# I'LL MAKE YOU BEAUTIFUL

# I'LL MAKE YO

## MAKEUP, HAIR, AND BEAUTY SECRETS

Photographer : MOSHE BRAKHA
Written By : MIJ SAVAGE
Illustrator : PAT IEMMITI
Designer : GAEL TOWEY
Art Director : ILANA HARKAVI

# U BEAUTIFUL

## FROM THE CREATOR OF *IL-MAKIAGE*

# ILANA HARKAVI

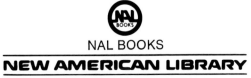

NAL BOOKS

**NEW AMERICAN LIBRARY**

NEW YORK AND SCARBOROUGH, ONTARIO

Having made my magic on a thousand faces, each one unique and each one beautiful, I have come to believe that the existence of beauty is part of a total creation we are all able to discover every day.

I give my sincere thanks to the Creator of all that beauty—and to the women who allowed me to use their faces as my canvas. Through time I have learned that we are all divine reflections of a single perfection.

NAL BOOKS TRADEMARK REG. U.S. PAT. OFF. AND FOREIGN COUNTRIES
REGISTERED TRADEMARK—MARCA REGISTRADA
HECHO EN CHICAGO, U.S.A.

SIGNET, SIGNET CLASSIC, MENTOR, ONYX, PLUME, MERIDIAN and NAL BOOKS are published in the United States by NAL Penguin Inc., 1633 Broadway, New York, New York 10019, in Canada by The New American Library of Canada Limited, 81 Mack Avenue, Scarborough, Ontario MIL IM8

Library of Congress Cataloging-in-Publication Data
Harkavi, Ilana.
  I'll make you beautiful.
  1. Beauty, Personal.    2.    Cosmetics.    3. Hairdressing.
I. Title
RA778.H235  1987     646.7'042     87–1532
ISBN 0-453-00555-1

First Printing, September, 1987

1 2 3 4 5 6 7 8 9

Printed in the United States of America

# TO MY DAUGHTER, AVIGAL

---

**To my husband and partner, Sam,** who together with me founded and realized the dream of *il-Makiage*. Thank you for sensing the perfect title: I'LL MAKE YOU BEAUTIFUL.

To my literary agent, Nancy Trichter, my editor, Barbara Lagowski, to Michaela Hamilton, Executive Editor of NAL, and my assistant, Linda Pedreira, my sincere gratitude.

To the modeling agencies—Elite, Ford, Legends, Nina Blanchard, and Mary Webb Davis—thank you for lending me all the beautiful faces.

# CONTENTS

Introduction  **viii**

## PART 1: THE MAKEUP LESSON 1

## PART 2: THE MANY LOOKS OF YOU 78

# INTRODUCTION

When an accident ended my first career—as a dancer—I was stunned and disappointed, but I was not confused. There was never any doubt in my mind as to what I would do next. For even as a child, exposed for the first time to the magical transformations that took place backstage, I had always been fascinated by makeup, by the shadings, textures, and colors that could turn actresses and dancers into whomever they wanted to be. And although friends tried to dissuade me, it was no use; after a period of formal study in cosmetics and an apprenticeship working behind the counter, I opened my own one-woman salon.

Now, nearly two decades later, I know that there are no "accidents." It was my destiny to indulge women's fantasies with color, to bring out their beauty with healthy natural cosmetics. But although I began less than twenty years ago, it might as well have been the dark ages. Color choices were incredibly limited (earth tones were "in" and everything else was nonexistent), cosmetics and hair colorings were by and large chemically based, and there was only a glimmer of consciousness about skin care. I felt as though I were working with one hand tied behind my back. I realized then that to bring my vision to other women I would have to create my own products, my own range of colors, an entire unlimited palette that could set women free to become anyone they wanted to be.

China Red, my first color, is still one of the most popular in the *il-Makiage* line. I followed with others: bright colors, muted colors, all the colors of the rainbow—and the palette gradually became limited only by my imagination. I reintroduced henna as a natural hair-coloring alternative to chemical dyes, and I brought it out in a range of shades, from sparkling blonde to deepest ebony. Soon Raquel Welch, Barbra Streisand, and hundreds of thousands of other women were using henna coloring. And I introduced henna gels and mousses for instant—and instantly washed away—hair coloring. It was *il-Makiage* that turned a writing tool—the pencil—into a versatile eye, cheek, and lip cosmetic (in forty shades!) and popularized kohl as a natural, hypoallergenic eye enhancer. Our highlighter dusts, glitter, iridescent shadows, and subtle mousse blushers enabled makeup artists to reach new heights in glamour, and the innovative collagen products I introduced to American women revolutionized skin care. And all of it—more than five hundred products—was the result of an "accident" that was somehow meant to be.

Now my *il-Makiage, Avigal,* and *Shoynear* lines of cosmetics and hair- and skin-care products are distributed in over one thousand stores worldwide. The client list of my salon encompasses a who's who of the fashion and entertainment worlds. I have been the recipient of numerous awards for my innovations (including the prestigious Nouvelle Esthètique Award in Paris for the top makeup artist of the year), and each season my advice about new trends is sought by beauty editors. Through the years I've worked with most of the top photographers, hairdressers, and stylists—and many of the most beautiful women in the world. I've run all around Europe and America with my makeup case. And now, the vision that I bring to the women who visit my salon is accessible to all.

But many women still don't know how to use the new world of makeup products and techniques. For years they've been feeling overwhelmed by its variety, by the sheer newness of it all. Many "experts" want to maintain the "mystery" of beauty as a world open only to its own select. And there has been no comprehensive guide to understanding today's makeup—until now.

I want to share the secrets of the salon with you. I want to teach you things you wouldn't learn even if you studied at the best beauty schools. I want you to envision yourself in a new way—alive with color and able to express all of your many moods and desires. I want to make *you* beautiful.

I've divided *I'll Make You Beautiful* into three parts in order to make it as simple and enjoyable as makeup has always been for me.

The first part, "The Makeup Lesson," is exactly that: In it I take you step-by-step through all the techniques, the tools, the makeup products you'll need to create a truly beautiful you. And I show you how to break the color barrier, enabling you to wear *any* color you like with dazzling results.

Do you need to put together a look in virtually no time flat? My five-minute makeup will get the freshest, most colorful you out the door in the wink of an eye. For a beautifully finished, long-lasting makeup, just let my eighteen easy steps be your guide. And if you want to take it to the limit, I will show you how to create a glamourous, state-of-the-art nighttime makeover with the very latest in makeup special effects. And all along the way, I'll let you in on the special tips I've learned in the nearly two decades I've spent making women beautiful.

Part 2, "The Many Looks of You," is your makeover dream come true. No other beauty book has ever gone beyond the traditional one-shot makeover to create the many faces of today's woman. In *this* innovative photographic section, I've taken nine top models from outdoor-fresh to office-chic, then on to the height of nighttime glamour. These breakthrough before, after, *after, after* makeovers illustrate makeup strategies for every season, every style, every mood imaginable. And with my hints, tips, and beauty secrets, you can achieve them all.

Part 3, "Beauty Basics," gets to the nitty-gritty and teaches you all you need to know about skin and body care, hair, and grooming. Included are my salon-tested, personalized skin programs, the *il-Makiage* minifacial, and special techniques to offset the effects of your monthly skin cycle. You'll learn to condition and color your hair with henna and finally, to put all the tips and techniques you've learned together in a revitalizing day of beauty.

There's so much to learn about beauty—whether I'm making up a celebrity like Diana Ross or Marlo Thomas, or giving a salon client a fresh look—I myself learn something new every day. What I hope this book will teach you is that you are unique—one of a kind—and in all that you do, all that you feel, and in every way you can imagine, you can be beautiful.

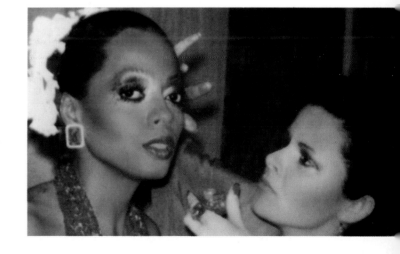

**"You have made me so beautiful,"** was Diana Ross's comment after I made her up in bold, glowing colors.

# PART I

# THE MAKEUP

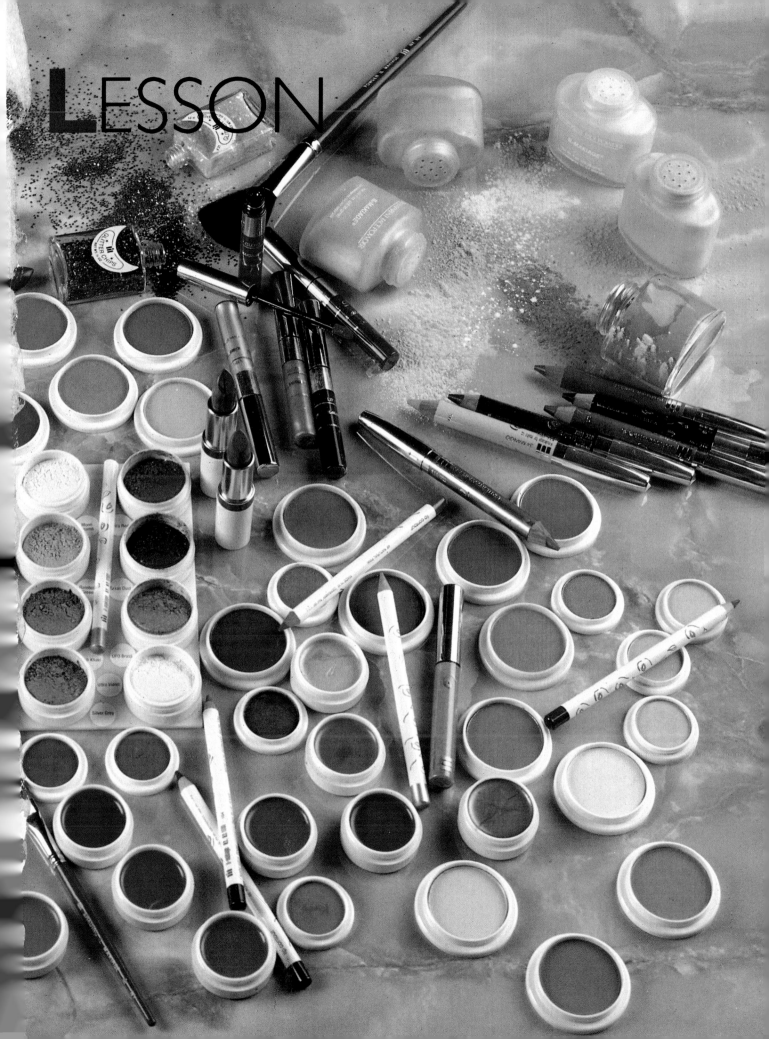

# LESSON

# Begin at the Beginning— You

The makeup lesson begins with its most important component—you. Every woman has something she loves about her face, some special feature that sets her apart from everyone else. Whether you're a famous model or the girl next door, when you walk into my salon I will always look for your special something.

The secret of enhancing a woman's beauty is in bringing out her best—the sensuous curve of her mouth, the expressive arch of her eyebrow, the soft, glowing color of her eyes. When I look at a woman's face and see the features that make her unique, I am taking the first step toward creating a more expressive, more exciting, more beautiful look. When you look in the mirror, focus on the features that will unlock your special beauty; they are the key to creating a more beautiful you.

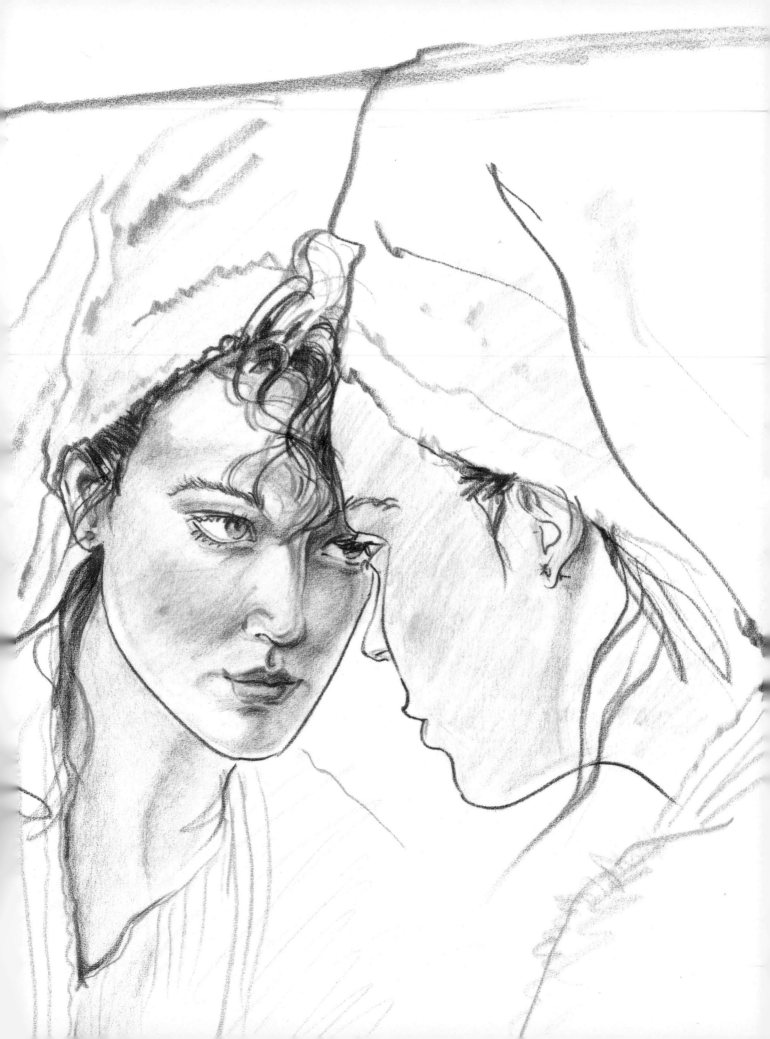

Before reaching for any cosmetics, take the time to consider the total you, the way you are now, today. If you believe, as I do, that *mood plus occasion equals change*, you know that tonight or tomorrow, next week or next month, you will be different.

In this modern world of ours, we all fulfill many different roles. Makeup can be a mirror to reflect those varied moods and activities. You may be an attractive, intelligent career woman by day, a chic girl-about-town by evening, and a sultry temptress by night. While the clean fresh look of your daytime makeup puts you at your best in the office, a shimmering, glowing, translucent makeup can light up those special evenings. Makeup can be the stuff of fantasy—its colors, textures, and sparkles will brighten any occasion. It can also be a communicator— of your moods, your personality, and your unique beauty.

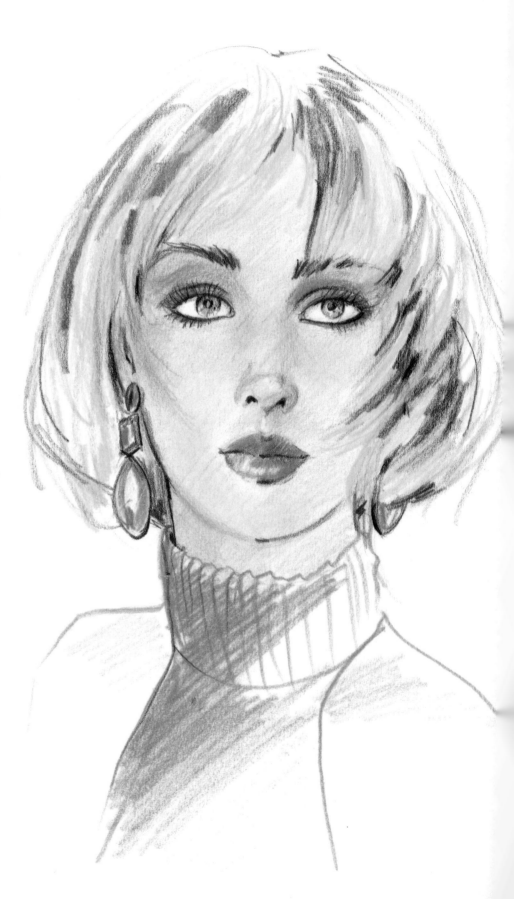

The right makeup can even change your mood. When you know you look good, you feel good, and every woman has experienced the feeling of confidence that comes from knowing she looks her best. On a recent television appearance I did a makeover on a young woman of thirty who felt all her good times were behind her. She had bleached blond hair and dark grayish-brown eyebrows; her skin was sallow and she wasn't wearing makeup; she couldn't even remember the last time she had cut her hair. Even her lovely hazel-green eyes were almost lost in her overall appearance. But I was sure I could make this woman beautiful. I deepened the color of her hair and lightened her eyebrows to match; an alabaster foundation took away the sallowness and gave her a beige skin tone; after reshaping her hair I gave her a pink-and-purple shaded makeup. The sheer pastels made her look radiant—they brought a spark to her beautiful eyes—she looked years younger and she felt marvelous. For half an hour after the show, she continued smiling at herself in the mirror.

*Every woman is beautiful:* You just have to know how to bring out your beauty. Perhaps someone told you what "type" you are, or how to key your makeup to the "seasonal" color palettes that have become a fad. But you're an individual, not a type, and your attitudes, priorities, and preferences are all yours, even if they change every day.

Don't allow the "experts" to tell you that pink is your color, you must never wear orange. You are far more complex than that. *You can wear any color.* But you must create a *total look.* For example: You recently went into a department store and tried a green eyeshadow. As you expected, it only reaffirmed your idea that green is your worst color. But you would have felt better about that green shadow if you had matched it with different accessories. Had you changed your pink lipstick to orange or brown, it would have been smashing. Had you replaced your blue earrings with gold, it would have made a perfect complement. And what color clothes were you wearing? What were the predominant shades of the rest of your makeup? If you didn't create a total look, you didn't give that green shadow a fair chance; you didn't give yourself a chance to break out of the color trap.

When I made up Marthe Keller for the movie *Black Sunday*, she was cast in the role of a terrorist. Here was a fair-skinned blonde, and she was playing a dark, dramatic Middle Easterner. I changed her hair color, used makeup to darken her light skin, and accented and deepened her eyes with a black kohl pencil. It worked—and if Marthe Keller could break all of the "experts'" color rules, so can you.

You want to express *your* personality in your makeup, and it's really not so difficult as many "experts" would have you believe. It's actually quite simple to make the woman you see in the mirror into anyone you want her to be. There are no rules to follow, only guidelines, and the proper techniques are easy to learn. Use your imagination, let yourself go; that's what makes makeup so much fun to play with—fun to choose, fun to apply, and fun to wear.

# BREAKING THE COLOR BARRIER

Recent advances in makeup technique can make today's woman look ten times better than her mother ever could. New makeup products provide an ease of application and a variety of textures and colors that would have been unimaginable to previous generations. The sheer, transparent, softly contoured and blended make-ups of the mid-eighties are not only the result of aesthetic choices, but of technical advances as well. Foundations are sheerer than ever before, enabling the skin to breathe. And *today's makeup is defined by color.*

To me, the burgeoning of color is one of the most exciting developments in the whole history of the art and science of makeup. When *il-Makiage* first introduced a new, broader color palette over a decade ago, the initial response by cosmetic counter sales personnel and popular books—by makeup professionals in general—

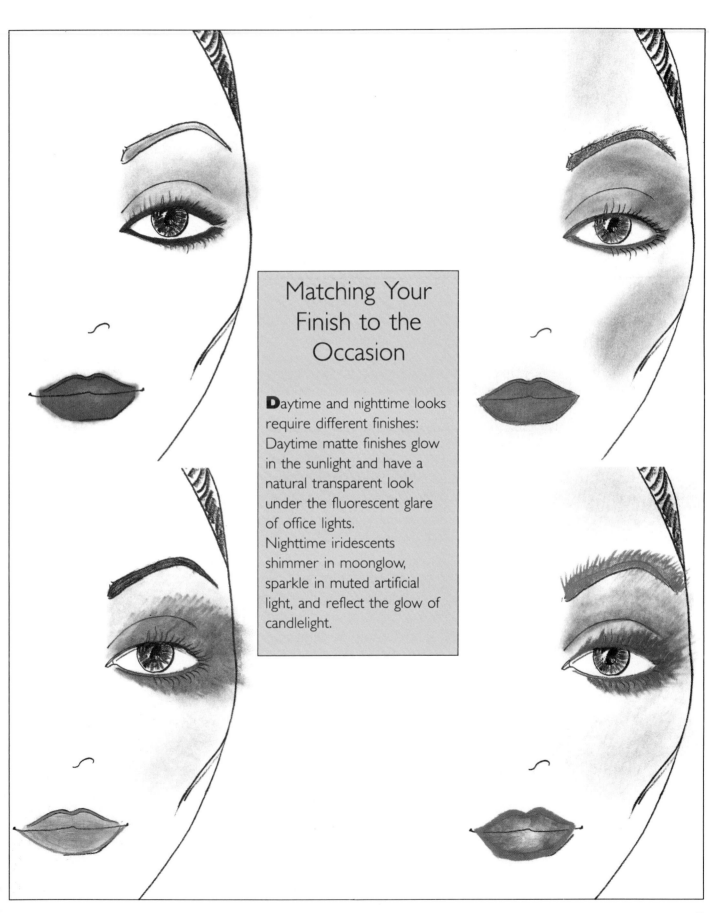

## Matching Your Finish to the Occasion

**D**aytime and nighttime looks require different finishes: Daytime matte finishes glow in the sunlight and have a natural transparent look under the fluorescent glare of office lights.
Nighttime iridescents shimmer in moonglow, sparkle in muted artificial light, and reflect the glow of candlelight.

was simplistic and limiting: Women were told to choose their cosmetics on the basis of their hair, skin, and eye color.

This idea might have seemed logical—but it was never really true. If you're not afraid, you can change your look as easily as I changed Marthe Keller's in *Black Sunday*. Try applying one of the new henna gels or mousses to change your hair color instantly (it washes right off the next time you shampoo); it will alter your natural coloring and expand your makeup options. Or start by combining new colors—the sparkling golds and muted magentas you love but never thought you could wear—with the blues and reds that you know look good on you. Little by little you'll find, as increasing numbers of women have found in the last few years, how using the entire range of colors can add excitement and glamour to your everyday looks as well as evening makeups.

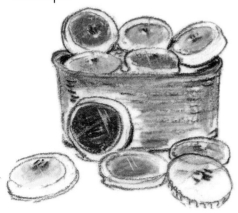

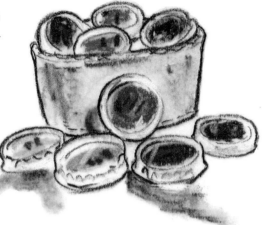

I know many women who have not spent their lives with makeup, as I have, still find the choices confusing, even intimidating. They may look at the muted purples and sparkling golds that are available to them, but they limit themselves to those "safe" shades they may have worn for years. To those women, color seems like a huge wall they can't get around and can't get over.

It's time for you to tear down the wall and *break the color barrier*. Remember, color makes you look good: It highlights your face, it enhances your mood, it helps bring out your best features. No matter what your age or coloration, you can wear transparent reds, pastels, or bolder, more intense colors; you can wear makeup with a flat matte or sparkling iridescent finish—or you can change from one color to another, one finish to another, depending on your mood and the occasion. Your choices are not really as confusing as they seem.

# **B**ASIC COLORS

Every woman can wear a wide variety of basic makeup colors: reds, blues, greens, browns and beiges, lavenders, whites, grays, and blacks. The basic colors will always work for you, while others may require skin preparation and matching with wardrobe and accessories to create a total look. But every one of these colors, under the right circumstances, can look great on anyone.

# **M**AKING COLOR WORK FOR YOU

Anybody can wear warm or cool color combinations, anybody can wear golds or silvers, blues or greens, pinks or oranges. Anybody can dazzle with color by coordinating to create a total look.

Just turn to the photos of Jade in "The Many Looks of You," Part 2 of this book for irrefutable evidence that coordination (and breaking the rules) can be a smashing success. Whereas the common wisdom of color limitation is that an Oriental woman with sallow skin can't possibly wear a silver makeup, I created a nighttime look for her that was based on silvers. Her look featured the interplay of opposites: The cold silvers and platinums in her makeup actually warmed up her sallow skin. Combined with a black suit and diamond-look earrings, the look was fabulous.

There are three simple guidelines to color coordination:

- Coordinate your makeup to a part of your natural coloring. A wine-colored blusher or lipstick will bring out the glow in auburn hair, for example; a blue shadow or mascara is a natural for a blue-eyed blonde.
- Coordinate your makeup shades to complement one another. Match your orange or brown lipstick with melons or peaches around your eyes and on your cheeks. Or do a makeup that consists entirely of iridescent silvers and lavenders—it's a fabulous nighttime look that's great even on people with naturally sallow complexions.

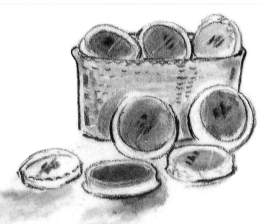

- Coordinate your makeup with your wardrobe and accessories; each will highlight the other. Decide what you're going to wear before you put on your lipstick, blusher, and eye makeup. A blue pencil will add an appropriate accent to your blue dress. Brass lipsticks and shadows will look great with that brown suit.

Think of that one accessory that will tie your total look together—a sea-green silk scarf, for example, to draw attention to eyes made up in complementary shades of shadow, pencil, and mascara. Don't wear your charcoal-and-pewter makeup with gold jewelry; they'll just detract from one another. Wear silver or turquoise earrings instead; I guarantee you'll look more pulled together.

You don't have to spend hours choosing color combinations; you can even do a great-looking two-minute one-color makeup as long as you remember to coordinate makeup with your wardrobe and accessories.

# Putting It All Together

Once you have an idea of the color combinations that work for you, you can venture farther afield, adding more and more of your creativity and personal style to the mix. To give you an idea of the possibilities, I've put together some of my favorite color combinations: one daytime look and one nighttime look for each hair and eye color. Match your coloring to the faces on the following pages for looks that will always work for you, but remember: With a little color coordination, every one of these combinations will look good—as part of a total look— on everyone.

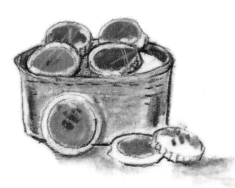

Alive with Color

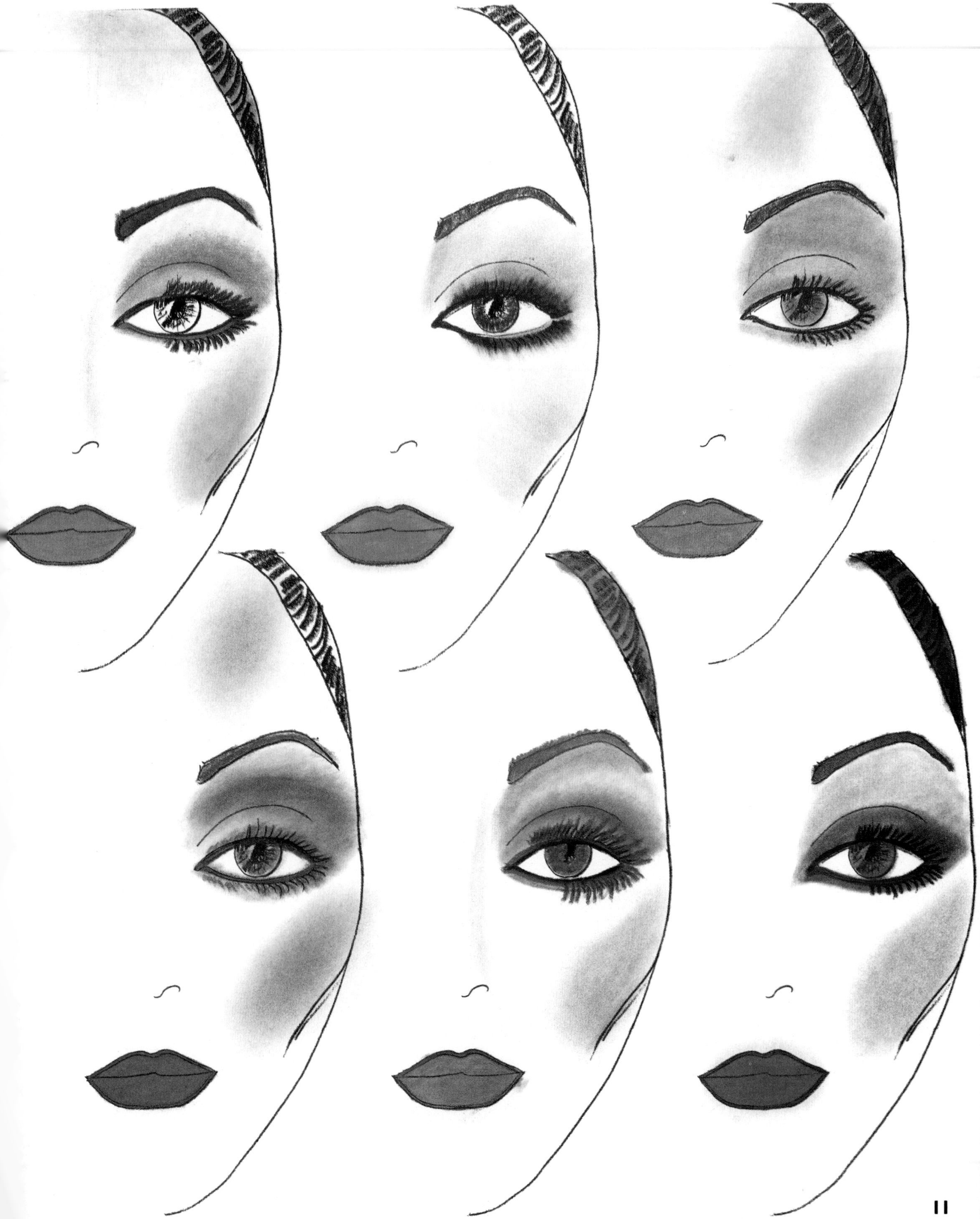

# CHAPTER THREE

# USING YOUR MAKEUP TOOLS

A woman's face is her canvas, and like any artist, you'll get more dramatic results when you use the right tools to apply foundations, shadows, gels, and mousse blushers. Fingerpainting is for children. Rubbing warm fingers on your skin opens up pores, which then drink up twice as much makeup as necessary. Fingers also spread foundation away from the center of your face, where you need the most coverage. And oil from fingers actually changes the consistency of your makeup.

Use the right tools to put on makeup—sponges, brushes, and applicators—and your application will be even, your blending imperceptible. You'll not only get better results than if you fingerpaint, you'll also have more fun.

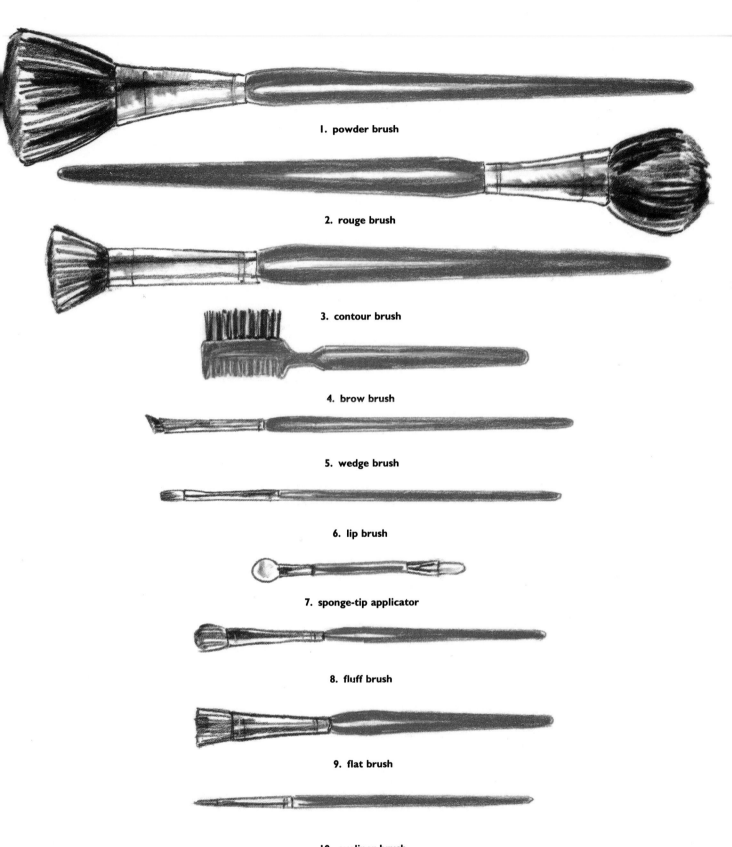

1. powder brush

2. rouge brush

3. contour brush

4. brow brush

5. wedge brush

6. lip brush

7. sponge-tip applicator

8. fluff brush

9. flat brush

10. eyeliner brush

# Essential Tools for Your Makeup Case

# MAKEUP SPONGES

Use a flexible makeup sponge to apply foundation as well as mousse and cream blushers. Thin, flat sponges are best because they don't absorb too much makeup. To increase flexibility, wash each sponge a few times before using. If you have sensitive skin, dip your sponge in alcohol to give it a softer touch. After use, wash the sponge in warm water and soap, and leave it to dry for the next day. Properly cared for, your sponge can last a year, and it gets better with use.

# MAKEUP BRUSHES

Brushes are invaluable tools for applying makeup. Their great variety and delicacy create innumerable possibilities for dramatic shading and subtle blending.

I recommend several different-sized brushes as standard equipment: one thick powder brush that can double as a blusher brush; a smaller contour brush to highlight and shade hard-to-reach areas around your nose and eyes; a thin brush to put on undereye concealer; a lip brush; and a small fluff brush to smooth on powder

shadows. Also useful, but hard to find, are small, wedge-shaped brushes that enable you to reach under bottom lashes or eyebrows. You can make your own by taking a small brush you don't often use and cutting the bristles on a slant. Of course, if your budget and imagination permit, you don't have to limit yourself to this selection— you'll definitely find use for others.

Good-quality brushes are fairly expensive but they're well worth the investment. A sable brush only gets better with time. Once it's been used and properly washed, it's more flexible than when new, and it can last forever.

Your brushes should be cleaned at least once every ten days. To loosen up the powders, dip in rubbing alcohol so that the alcohol covers the hairs of the

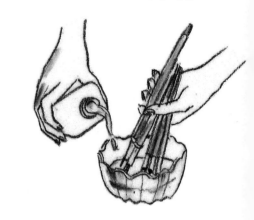

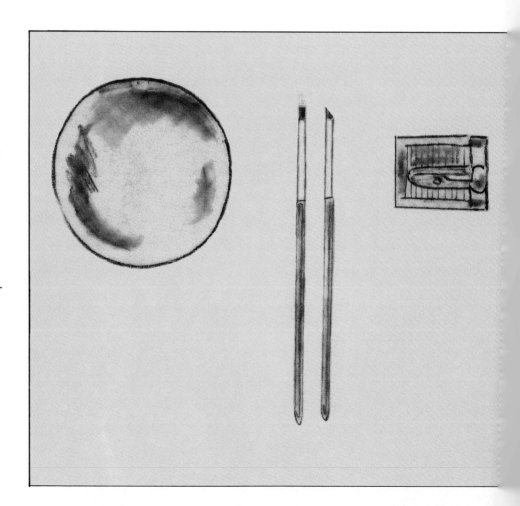

brush (not the metal). Touch the hairs against the side of the bowl and let the liquid run off. Place on a towel or tissue to dry overnight.

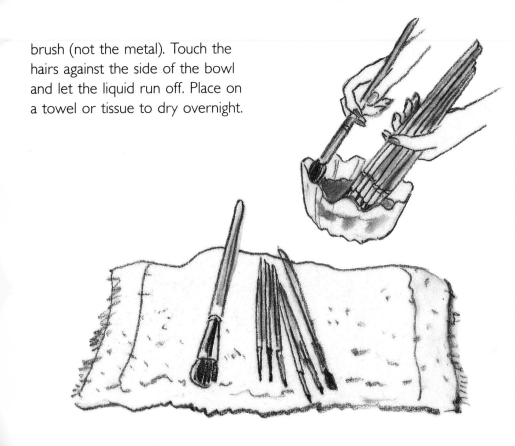

# SPONGE-TIP APPLICATORS

Applicators are excellent for applying iridescent shadows; the sponge tips hold iridescence extremely well and don't allow the shadows to flake over your face. Use a sponge applicator tip if you desire a more intense color than the sheer finish a sable brush will give you. I use a wide, flat sponge applicator to sweep color under eyebrows and a thin, rounded tip to apply shadow under bottom lashes. Sponge tips are also great for blending pencil lines into shadows.

Wash your applicators gently in soap and water after using.

# EYELASH CURLER

Most people know that one of the keys to beautiful eyes is to widen them, but few people realize that an eyelash curler is *the* indispensable tool for doing it. Even though you use your eyelash curler before you put on mascara, makeup residue that sometimes clings to lashes can make the curler stick. Clean it regularly to prevent mascara buildup.

Now that you've got your tools in place, you're ready to move on!

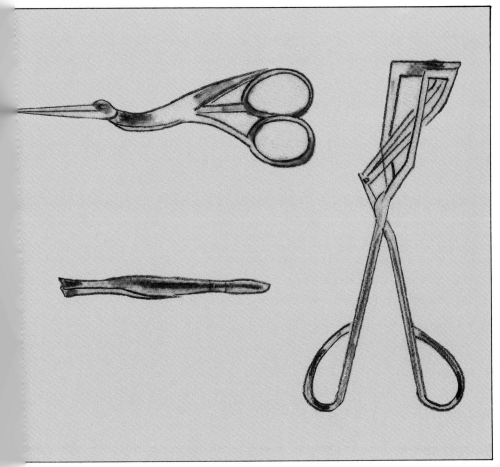

# **P**REPARING **Y**OUR **F**ACE FOR **C**OLOR

The other day an eager new customer came into *il-Makiage*; she was very anxious to try one of the new shades of mousse blender I had put on display. We chose a shade that was perfect for her, but when I applied it pink patches appeared on her face. Because she hadn't bothered to put on either foundation or moisturizer, the blusher stuck directly to her skin and the beautiful, colorful makeup we could have created was blotchy right from the beginning.

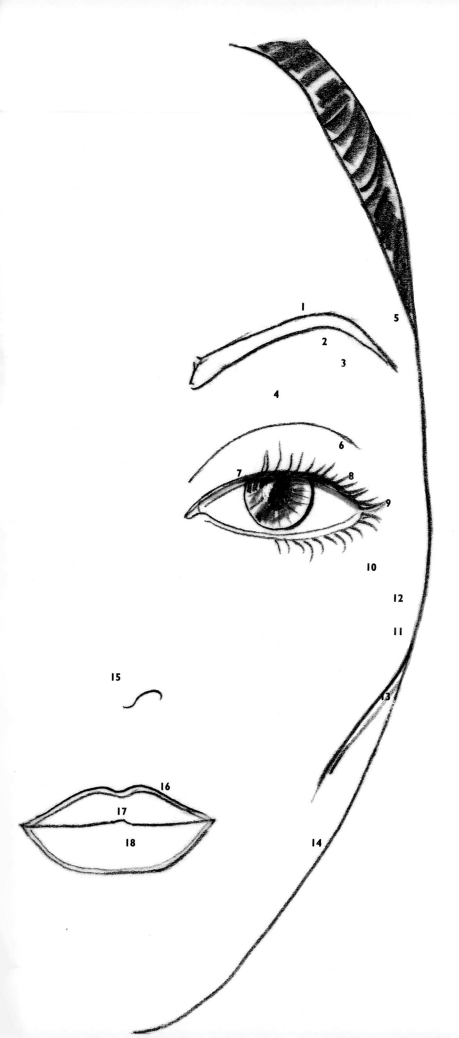

## il-Makiage Face Chart

1. EYEBROW _____
2. EYE (HIGHLIGHT) _____
3. BROW BONE _____
4. EYELID (BASE) _____
5. TEMPLES (CONTOUR) _____
6. EYE (CONTOUR) _____
7. INNER CORNER_____
8. OUTER CORNER _____
9. EYELINER _____
10. CHEEKBONE
    (HIGHLIGHT) _____
11. CHEEKBONE
    (HIGHLIGHT) _____
12. OVER CHEEKBONE AREA
    (BLUSHER) _____
13. UNDER CHEEKBONE AREA
    (CONTOUR) _____
14. JAWLINE (CONTOUR) _____
15. NOSE (HIGHLIGHT) _____
        (CONTOUR) _____
16. LIP OUTLINE _____
17. LIPSTICK _____
18. LIPGLOSS OR
    HIGHLIGHT _____

# FIRST THINGS FIRST— **M**OISTURIZER

Moisturizer is exactly what the name suggests: a product that keeps skin moist and protects it from the ravages of the environment. If your skin is normal, dry, or, like most people's, mixed or combination (part dry and part normal or part normal and part oily), you need moisturizer before you put on your makeup. Without it, any part of your face that lacks moisture will resist color, and expression lines and imperfections in your skin will only be accentuated.

For most women, I suggest using a moisturizer every morning regardless of whether you're planning to wear makeup. It seals your skin, preparing it for a long-lasting makeup and protecting your pores from dirt, dust, hot sun, cold wind—even your own fingers.

## Choosing a Moisturizer

There are moisturizers specially formulated for each skin type. Generally speaking, the oilier your complexion, the higher the percentage of alcohol your moisturizer should contain. But you don't have to look at the ingredients on the label to know which product you need; you just need to know your skin type. If you don't know yours, turn to page 150 for a simple test you can do yourself.

## Using a Moisturizer

The first thing to remember about using moisturizer is to use it sparingly. Here's a step-by-step illustrated guide to keeping your skin soft and moist without clogging pores.

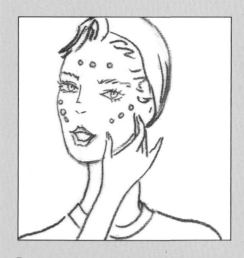

**1.** Squeeze a small amount of moisturizer onto the back of one hand.

Apply in a three-dot pattern (three dots on either cheek, on either side of your neck, and across the forehead).

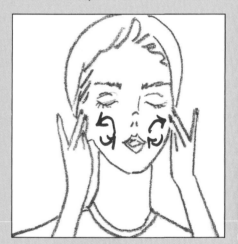

**5.** Massage the cheeks, chin, and nose with the balls of your fingers, using light circular motions.

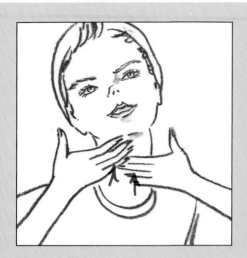

**2.** Gently stroke your neck with alternating hands in an upward direction.

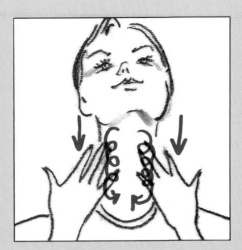

**3.** Using the two middle fingers of each hand, blend down the neck in a circular motion.

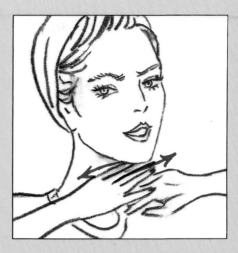

**4.** With the backs of your fingers, vigorously massage under your chin in a side-to-side motion.

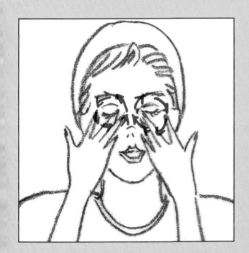

**6.** Massage lightly up and around eyes.

Gently press the pressure points at the outer ridge of the eyebone.

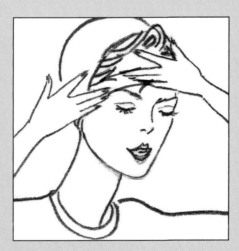

**7.** Stroke the forehead back and forth as though you were smoothing away worry lines.

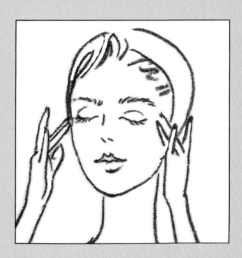

**8.** Lightly tap your fingers up and around your eyes several times.

Place a dot of moisturizer at the corners of your lips.

Lightly tap around lips, blending moisturizer in.

Once your skin is properly moisturized, you're ready for makeup.

## Protecting Naturally Moist Skins

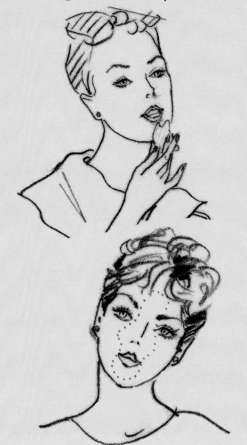

### FOR OILY SKIN

**Y**ou probably don't need a moisturizer, particularly if you are acne-prone. But please don't put your powders and blushers directly on blemished or problem skin. Before putting on makeup, clean your face with an astringent lotion (which removes excess oils, disinfects, and helps keep your skin dry), and use a drying lotion (which helps dry out blemishes) under your foundation. The combination will keep your sensitive skin clean and infection-free.

### FOR MIXED SKIN TYPES

**P**ut moisturizer only where you need it. If you have oily/normal combination skin, concentrate moisturizer on the side of your face (your cheeks, jawline, temples). Clean oily areas (particularly the forehead, nose, and chin "T-zone") with astringent lotion before applying your foundation.

If you have dry/normal combination skin, use moisturizer everywhere, but use less on your T-zone.

### THE SUNSCREEN MOISTURIZER OPTION

**I**f you have normal, dry, or mixed skin, you can use sunscreen anytime as a quick and easy greaseless moisturizer. If your skin is oily, you can still use sunscreen, but use it very sparingly.

# CAN YOU KEEP A SECRET?— **C**ONCEALERS

How important is concealer to me? I leave the house in the morning with just my concealer and lipstick, confident that with only these two products I can do a full makeup.

Concealer lightens dark circles under the eyes, covers sunspots and minor blemishes, and softens expression lines. The *il-Makiage* concealer is called "TV Touch," because it's effective even under the glare of the lights, where even the smallest imperfection shows.

I take my concealer compact wherever I go. And I use it *every time I do a makeup*—even on a twenty-year-old model who thinks she's much too young to have anything to hide. But you can be twenty and meticulous about your sleeping habits and still have a dark circle under your eye; the skin that surrounds the eye is extremely fragile, and it is visibly darker than the surrounding skin on almost everyone's face. Your foundation won't cover up shadows; and adding color will only emphasize them. But if you blend concealer under your sleepy-looking eyes your whole face will brighten up.

## Choosing a Concealer

Concealers come in small pots, tubes, or in compacts that you can carry around with you easily. In order to lighten dark, shadowy skin to match the rest of your face, you should choose a concealer a shade or two lighter than your predominant skin tone.

## Using a Concealer

Apply your concealer before you smooth on foundation. It will blend into your foundation and disappear once you've dabbed your makeup sponge over it.

Before applying concealer, first check the undereye area so that you'll know exactly where the shadowy area begins and ends. *Don't put concealer where you don't need it.* If you put it all around your eyes, you'll trap it in your smile lines and lose some of its anti-aging effect.

# LASTING COLOR STARTS WITH FOUNDATION

What does foundation do for you? The *right* foundation will even out the color of your skin, remove minor imperfections from view, and provide you with a smooth, clean base upon which to build any makeup look you wish. It is also, like moisturizer, a layer of protection from the environment. And it's an absolute essential if you want a makeup that will look colorful and last all day.

## Matching Foundation to Your Skin Type

There are several different types of foundation to choose from; how do you select the one which is best for you? Principally, by determining your skin type and choosing a product formulated to enhance your skin's health and condition.

**Water-based foundations** are good for skin that is still full of natural moisture. You can usually find separate formulations for your own naturally moist skin type—whether it's oily or mixed. Water-based foundations are easy to work with and have a sheer finish.

**"Medicated" foundations** are water-based foundations especially designed for oily or acne-problem skin. (The term "medicated" is used by skin-care specialists but won't appear on the label because of FDA regulations.) Medicated foundations are even more watery in consistency than regular water-based foundations; they can sometimes be distinguished (in the absence of labeling) by the way they separate into liquid and

semisolid components when left standing. This type of foundation has a light finish, but its good coverage will prove invaluable as a protection against blemishes. Use an astringent lotion first to cut down on your natural oiliness.

**Liquid oil-based foundations** are designed for dry skin. Their oily texture gives a more glowing finish, which is desirable when you have skin that's on the dry side. Their coverage is generally better and longer-lasting than water-based formulations for this type of complexion.

Oil-based foundations are also suitable for skin that is temporarily dehydrated and can't take the potentially drying effects of a water-based foundation. But they are not recommended for oily or acne-prone skin; the lanolin, glycerin acids, or mineral oils they contain will only encourage the spread of blemishes.

**Cream foundations** (whipped cream and matte cream) and *makeup sticks* contain a fairly high proportion of mineral oil. They're very good protection for dry and sensitive skin, as they have extra moisturizing agents in them. The cream also penetrates, moisturizes, and covers expression lines.

## Matching Foundation to Skin Tone

Foundation shades range from very light porcelain through the all-important beiges down to dark tans and bronzes. As you know I love color; it's exciting and it's fun. You can experiment with color— you can wear any color shadow or rouge—but please, except under special circumstances, don't experiment with the color of your foundation. Why not? Here's an example:

Suppose you want your skin to appear as though you've just returned from a Caribbean vacation; you choose a foundation color several shades darker than your natural skin tones. Your borrowed "tan" will never really look like your skin at all—worse yet, it highlights rather than hides all the expression lines around your eyes and mouth. With the wrong color foundation, no one will look at your beautiful lips and colorful eyes—just at your wrinkles.

So if you're tempted to add color by buying an instant tan, or a glowing pink or some other "fantasy" shade of foundation, re-member—you can add plenty of color with the cosmetics you put on over your foundation. But the colors of blusher, shadow, lipstick, and pencils won't look right unless your foundation is matched as closely as possible to your skin color.

I've looked at a lot of faces over the years, and believe me, I know how difficult it is to fit skin colors into neat categories: A fair complexion may have more beige in it than pink or white, and a black skin may actually have a warm orange tone. (Diana Ross is so scrupulous about matching her foundation color to her skin that I always carefully mix two colors of foundation together for her, to get it just right.) Skin color can change as well: I've seen many older women who haven't changed their foundation shade for years, but whose skin has lost color and who now have freckles and sunspots —and who therefore need a new foundation.

## The Important Moment— Choosing a Foundation

Since I want you to look as beau-tiful as you can be, I'm asking you to throw out your preconceived ideas about the "right" shade for you. The next time you buy foun-dation, start from scratch. Try the sample bottles available to you at the cosmetics counter; you can al-ways return to your old shade if it really is right for you.

You know how important it is to match foundation shades as closely as possible to skin tones. But how do you choose? Your face is never entirely consistent in color; it varies in tone from fea-ture to feature, from your cheek-bones, which catch a great deal of the sun's direct rays, to the hol-lows, which are naturally shaded. And you have only to hold your hand up next to your face when you look in the mirror to see the disadvantages of using the back of your hand to test a foundation shade. I know of only *one foolproof method for matching foundation to skin tone:* Put a drop or two *on your neck,* rub it in, and see how it blends with your skin. The skin on your neck is the same color as the skin on your face, but without po-tentially confusing variations in color. Once you have found a shade that matches the color of your neck, you have found the right foundation shade for you.

## Using Foundation

Here's a general rule of thumb about putting on makeup; it most definitely applies to foundation: *The less you apply, the longer it lasts and the better it looks.* And the proper tool for putting on foundation is your *makeup sponge.*

With a little bit of practice, putting on foundation will take you a minute, or even less. Here's how.

Fold your sponge between your fingers to increase control. Put a few drops of foundation onto the fold of the sponge. Distribute foundation in a "three-dot" pattern: three dots of foundation on each cheek, three across the forehead, two on the nose, and one on the chin.

Still keeping your sponge folded, blend foundation onto your skin. Work in long, even strokes down to the jawline and up to the hairline until the cheeks and forehead take on an even tone. (If you've chosen the right shade, you don't need any foundation at all on your neck. Since it tends to soil collars, I avoid it completely unless I want to show off a low-cut neckline, or for a "special effect" nighttime makeup.)

Then turn your attention to the hard-to-reach areas around your nose, mouth, and chin. *Dab*—don't rub—with a corner of your sponge, until these areas are well covered.

Finally, blend your foundation into your lips and apply one more dot to each eyelid. Stroke the skin around the eye gently, working the foundation inward without pulling the lids. This fragile skin can stretch and wrinkle if not handled with care.

*Putting foundation over eyelids and lips is the first step toward creating long-lasting eye and lip makeups.*

## Skin That Doesn't Take Color

Certain colors "turn" or change when applied to sallow—or yellow-toned—skin. Yellows, greens, and oranges can look like mud; pinks and peaches can accentuate a "tired" look and make skin look washed out. *But take heart: You can break the color barrier.*

If your skin is slightly yellow (just enough to resist taking colors), you'll need an alabaster foundation as close as possible to your natural skin tones. That was the solution for one of my clients, a seventeen-year-old model with ash-brown hair and beautiful, smooth (but slightly sallow) skin. Once we neutralized the yellow with a beige foundation, we were able to put on a fresh daytime makeup of pinks and peaches. Later, we gave her a makeup that featured a previously unwearable orange with a gold accent. Her skin held the colors beautifully—and it looked alive.

Check coverage before applying the rest of your makeup. The color and texture should be light and even. Then dab any large pores of small imperfections with your sponge until they disappear. Finally, blot with a tissue to remove any excess.

## You Might Need a Toner

Some skin types respond to a slight change of foundation shade. But some of you may need to do more; that's when I recommend a skin toner. A toner is a sort of liquid foundation that acts as a primer for your foundation.

Use a toner only if you absolutely can't do without one, like the young woman who recently came into the salon with skin so flushed it looked as if it were on fire. Her skin color simply overwhelmed many makeup colors—pinks, oranges, anything with even a hint of red. Of course, I couldn't let her out of the salon until I had solved her problem by applying a green toner under her foundation. Most of the fiery redness disappeared under the toner, the rest under her foundation. For the first time in her life, she broke her own personal color barrier.

If you have olive-toned Mediterranean or Oriental skin, you need a beige foundation close to your skin tones to offset the sallowness. If your sallow skin can't be corrected by beige foundation, try a violet toner. The violet will

## Summertime Foundation Options

**S**unscreen is not only a moisturizer option. It can also be a fine makeup base for an informal summer makeup.

The secret to creating a fresh, lively, sunscreen-based makeup is to put as little as possible over it while still adding color. When using a sunscreen as a makeup base, I favor cream- or mousse-based cosmetics because they go on smoothly over the sunscreen and protect eyes and cheeks.

Because your summer skin has more color, you can use lighter makeup colors to go over your usual base. There will be times you will want to wear stronger colors, but what about trying a pale pink blush or bronze transparent powder for a change? Or pinks and yellows or greens for eyeshadows? These are "summery" colors that can look wonderful over your usual foundation and more colorful summer skin. (Conversely, you may want to warm up your paler winter skin by putting stronger colors over your foundation: deeper pinks or blues, earthy brown lipsticks and shadows, and warm blusher shades.)

If you tan heavily, you can either change your foundation shade from season to season, or you can use a tinted moisturizer as a one-step summertime moisturizer and foundation. The slight pigment in the tinted moisturizer evens out the color of your newly tanned skin, and sun-dried skin can certainly use the extra moisture it provides. If you have dry, normal, or combination skin, you can use tinted moisturizer with the same colorful makeups you normally use.

give your skin a flattering beige tone, and you will be able to wear new colors like yellows and greens that look so fresh and summery on other people but have always looked so washed-out on you.

If your black skin has an ashen look to it, you require a wine shade of toner. It will give ashen-looking skin a warm, earthy tone.

If you have patches of uneven skin (flushed or marked by large sunspots or patches of dark pigmentation) you'll need a white toner under your foundation.

**This summer makeup can be created with a sunscreen (applied by sponge), lip gloss, an eye pencil (used on brows and as a lip accent), and a pale-colored cream shadow put right over the crease of the eyes for a sensational finish.**

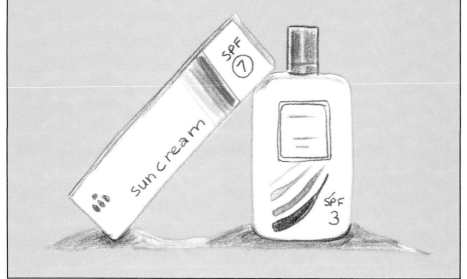

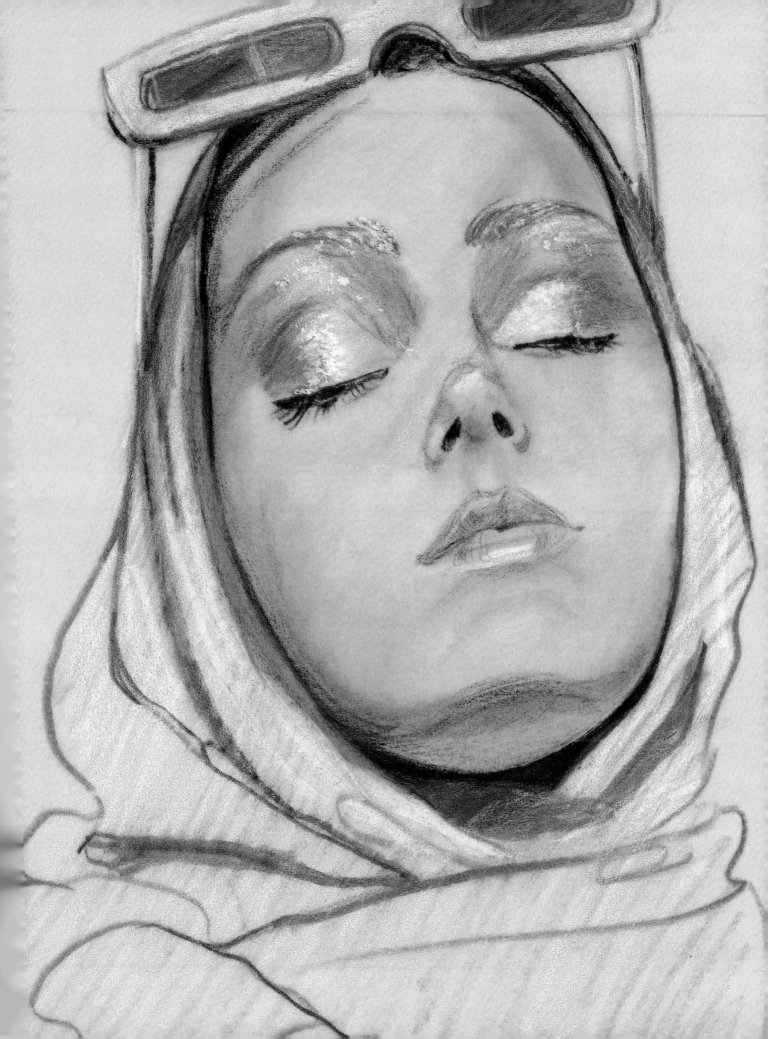

# SETTING YOUR BASE— TRANSPARENT POWDER

Loose transparent powder whisked on by a big powder brush sets your makeup base by removing the oiliness that rises to the surface of the skin after you have put on moisturizer and foundation. Once you have set your makeup base with powder, your blusher, shadows, and lipsticks will go on smooth. Nor will you have to worry about blotchiness. A final dusting with colored powder after you have completed putting on your colorful cosmetics will set your entire look and give it a light, sheer finish.

## Choosing a Powder

In general, I prefer a powder shade that is matched as closely as possible to your foundation. But if your skin is extremely pale, you may compensate by using a loose transparent powder a shade darker than your foundation. Because of the transparency of the powder the results will look completely natural.

## Using Powder

Think of your powder brush as a feather in your hand; dab lightly and your powder will be ab-

sorbed perfectly into your foundation, thus enabling it to absorb natural oils before they break through to the surface.

Dab over cheeks, chin, nose, and forehead. If you brush rather than dab, your powder will "drift" and create a heavy look, not the matte finish you desire. But do brush powder over eyelids and lips; this will help ensure that your lip and eye makeups will be as long-lasting as your rouges.

Use more powder if you have oily skin, less if your skin tends toward dryness (powder makes the skin dryer). If you find that even after dabbing on powder you get oily patches over your nose, chin, and forehead, pat your brush along your T-zone, or wherever oily patches are a problem, until all the powder has been absorbed.

Loose powder and this simple dabbing technique will give you a far better and longer-lasting finish than you could ever achieve with a powder puff and a compact. But don't throw your compact away. I always carry one in my purse for touchups. It's fast and convenient, and as long as you wipe away excess oiliness with a tissue before using pressed powder you won't have the problem of your powder puff picking up oil. And if you're not using foundation, pressed powder gives more coverage than loose powder. It won't last as long as foundation and loose powder as it sits on

top of the skin, but it is an alternative, particularly when you need to do a fast makeup.

Some people prefer using tissues to apply powder; I urge you only to use them to blot away excess oiliness. Tissues are made of wood fiber: They're scratchy, inflexible, and absorbent, and will waste a tremendous amount of powder.

# ADDING DIMENSION— CONTOURING

Your face is three-dimensional: rounded here, flatter elsewhere; composed of curves, angles, and hollows—more like the subject of a sculpture than a painting. But Mother Nature doesn't always use as delicate a hand as did an artist like Degas, and you may want to create illusions to perfect her handiwork.

*Contour creates the illusion of a perfectly shaped face and features through the use of shadows.* It is an optional step in your everyday makeup, and although you will probably not use it when you put on a quick makeup before you go to the office in the morning, you will want to know its principles, for they are essential in creating the more sophisticated makeup looks that will light up your evenings and special events.

Your eye is always attracted to light, and so it is with makeup as well: Light shades accentuate and bring your features forward; dark shades deemphasize and diminish them. And that simple and logical principle is the basis of contouring.

Place a light high above your mirror and take a look at your face: Your brow bones, your cheekbones, the bridge of your nose, and your chin catch the light; the hollow of your cheeks, your eye sockets, and the area underneath your lower lip are thrown into darkness. These lights and darks are the clues by which your eye recognizes the natural contours of your facial features. When you shape your face with makeup you may emphasize them or you may seek to change them—but you will always use the same principles of light and dark by which you recognize them.

## Choosing a Contour Shade

Use brown makeup shades to contour under rouge—shades that create the shadows that, in turn, create illusion. Don't worry, you are not throwing your face into darkness; you will be adding contrast—your lighter, brighter makeup—later.

Generally and simply stated, the shade of brown you choose will depend on the color of your hair. If your hair is red, or brown with red or gold tones in it, you will choose a contour color that's a light brown with a red or gold accent. If you have blond, ash-brown, or black hair with no red highlights, choose an ash-brown (brown with gray) shade of contour.

## How to Contour

The same basic technique applies wherever you use contouring; under your cheeks, your jaw, your nose, or your forehead. First, brush contour powder over the area you wish to shadow. (Always use less makeup, rather than more, when you're in doubt about how much to apply.) Blend well (in a generally downward direction), until the line has become a shadow. The area you have contoured will recede in relation to the brighter areas surrounding it.

## Working with Your Cheekbones

Your cheekbones are the anchor of your facial structure; they provide interest and dimension to the entire facial plane. If you want your face to have structure, don't hide your cheekbones. If you are still in your teens you may have a little extra fullness around your jawline, which will disappear in time, but in the meantime you will want to create a more definite structure for your face. *Once you have learned to work with your cheekbones you will bring structure to your otherwise potentially unstructured appearance.*

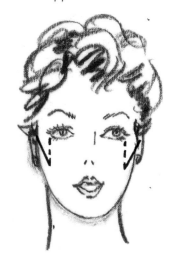

But to work with your cheekbones you must first find them. A good method is to hold your finger at the outer corner of your eye and trace an imaginary line straight down until you reach the bone directly below. Now move your finger diagonally up and out to the top of your ear. That's the course of your cheekbone. Keep it in mind whenever you contour your face (and later as well, when you add the first blush of makeup color—rouge).

# Creating the Perfect-Shaped Face

**A**n oval-shaped face is generally considered to be perfect because it is so well balanced. In the oval-shaped face, the distance from hairline to eyebrow equals that from the cheekbone to the jawline. Lift your hair off your face and look in the mirror to see how your face shape deviates from this perfect symmetry. If your face is not oval (and most aren't), you can create the illusion through the use of contour.

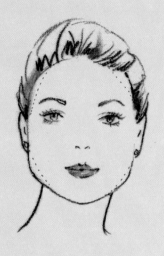

**Square**

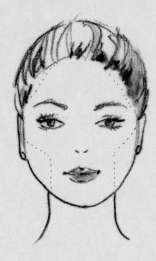

**Round**

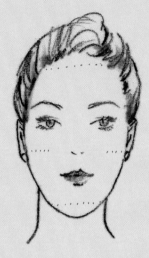

**Long**

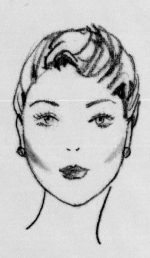

**Oval**

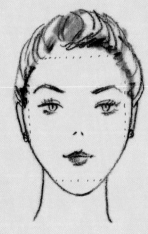

**Triangle**

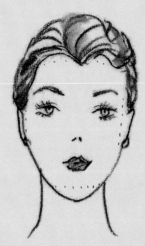

**Heart**

*To shorten a long face:* To increase width, blend contour straight across from the middle of your cheekbone (even with the pupil of your eye) directly outward to the top of your ear; to shorten your forehead, place contour directly across your hairline; to shorten your chin, apply contour *over* your chin and jawline.

*To narrow a round face:* Working from the bottom up, blend contour along the side of your jaw; from under your cheekbone diagonally up to the tip of your ear; from the top of your ear to your temple. To further create the illusion of a more slender face, narrow your nose by contouring the sides along the nostrils.

## Creating More-Perfect Features

You may wish to alter various features through contouring, either to minimize areas you wish to hide or to maximize those you want to show off.

**To show off a long neck:** Lightly blend contour straight down the sides of your neck from your ear. This will also narrow and lengthen a wide neck.

**To hide a double chin:** Add your brown contour shade as a shadow under your chin.

**To minimize a wide jawline:** Use contour over the jawbone to shadow and narrow it.

**To narrow a wide nose:** Use contour along the sides of your nose, leaving the center open.

**To widen a narrow nose:** Apply your brown contour shade directly down the center of your nose and leave the sides bare.

**To make your nose more uplifted:** Add contour under your nose in the area of your nostrils.

**To recede a prominent bridge:** Use brown contour directly on the bridge and add a contrasting white below to draw attention away.

**To lower a high forehead:** Blend contour shade directly across your hairline.

**To round and narrow a wide forehead:** Apply contour at the temples.

**To minimize fleshy eyelids:** Use contour along the bone line of the brow (not in the crease, where you will use a lighter shade). This will open your eye and recede the fleshiness of your lids.

There are, of course, many other possible uses of contour. And like the above, most of them are simple common sense, as long as you remember—dark recedes, light emphasizes.

# A BEAUTIFUL, COLORFUL YOU

The techniques of preparation for color are simple, and the few moments you take to get your face ready soon fly by, with results that are well worth the time. Once you have applied your moisturizer, concealer, foundation, transparent powder, and, if you wish, contour, your face is ready to take color—fabulous, glorious color.

Blush on blusher for cheeks that glow; blend in infinite combinations of shadow and pencil for mysterious or playful or sexy eyes; stroke on lipstick or gloss and let your lips say whatever you want them to; add a colored powder to bring it all together. Morning, noon, or night, the colorful makeups you wear highlight your best features and bring light to your face. Color transforms makeup into self-expression.

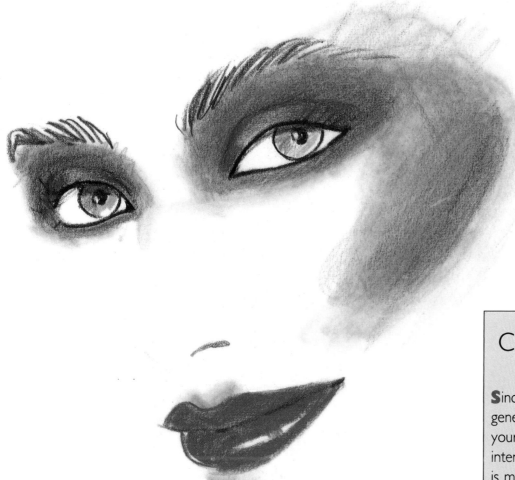

## Cheeks that Glow

**S**ince the sun's rays (and light in general) hit different areas of your face with more or less intensity, the skin in some places is more highly colored than in others. Light catches the cheekbones first, so you need less color over them and more under them to accent your cheekbones and define your facial structure. A soft, eye-catching glow that enhances the curve of your cheek is exactly the look you want from your blusher.

# THE FIRST BLUSH OF COLOR— ROUGE

Rouge, or blusher, is the first light on your face, your first touch of color. It is also a quick and easy way to add definition to your face, for it is applied in the all-important area directly underneath your cheekbones.

## Choosing a Blusher

Powder and cream blushers are the classic rouges. Fast-working mousses and gels have recently gained considerable popularity as well. Other cosmetics, not specifically designed as rouges (pencils, for example), can also be used, particularly as highlighters. With such a wealth of products available, before you buy your next blusher you will want to find the ones that best suit your skin type and makeup requirements.

**Flat matte powder blushers** are excellent for more formal makeup moods (unless you have very dry skin); applied over moisturizer, or better yet, moisturizer and foundation, they give marvelous, lasting color. And since they are applied with a brush and don't rapidly change in texture, you can put them on slowly, a trace at a time, until you are completely satisfied with the results.

**Powder iridescents** are good for most skin types when used over moisturizer and foundation. Their sparkle is most appropriate for evening special effects, but beware: Iridescent cosmetics get their glowy color from ground fish scales, which can irritate sensitive skin.

**Cream blushers** are designed for women with dry skin. They are rich in emollients and glide on easily when applied with a makeup sponge.

**Mousses** are good for all skin types. They are light in texture, go on like a cream, and dry to a very long-lasting powder finish. Once you get used to applying and blending very quickly with your sponge, you and your "mousse" can go anywhere, from gym to office to dinner out— almost instantaneously. I'm really very enthusiastic about mousses for their exceptionally quick, extraordinarily colorful finish.

**Gels** are suitable for those lucky enough to have unblemished skins; blended in quickly with your sponge they give your cheeks a glow, a sheer finish, and relatively minimal coverage. As with a mousse, gels dry fast, so you must work fast.

## Choosing Blusher Colors

I predict that you will find one basic blusher—the color that best complements your hair and skin tones—that you'll feel so comfortable with you'll reach for it morning after morning, before you've even decided on your wardrobe or your other makeup for the day. But you will be missing something if you become so attached to it that you ignore the other basic blusher colors. In many cases, teamed with lipstick and shadows, rouges other than your standard can create a smashing look.

There are many basic colors you may resist because you are simply unused to them; for example, the magentas and some of the other definite deep pinks. A few years ago colors like magenta didn't even exist, but in the past year I've put magenta on more people than I can count, and it invariably looks good.

When you see a color that you like but are afraid to use because it seems too colorful, bear in mind that it will look much softer once you have fully blended it in. And you really can't tell the true effect of your rouge until you've finished the rest of your makeup. Particularly when I'm working with one of the lighter shades, I often find myself adding more at the end of a makeup because it suddenly looks pallid alongside my shadow and lipstick.

You may also choose a blusher to match your clothes. I recently did a demonstration using as my model a friend who generally doesn't wear very much makeup. Fitting the makeup to her personality and taste, I decided on a quiet look, using as my theme blushers and shadows that matched the very pretty mauve jacket she was wearing. The mauve rouge I chose blended in so softly that I was able to put on a brighter pink lipstick and still keep the soft understated look of the makeup.

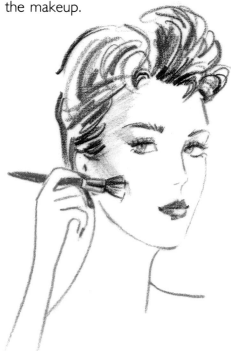

If you wish, you can be more adventurous with your blusher color, choosing, for example, a lilac or a yellow. These are among the colors that look terribly exotic when you see them in a palette but can be beautiful when blended into your skin.

## When You Make a Mistake

When you make a mistake applying blusher (and everyone does, even the professionals), you will end up with a terrible mess if you start rubbing at the area with tissues or try to wash the mistake away with a wet makeup sponge. The professional way to deal with mistakes (and the one that causes the least grief) is to brush a pale shade of ivory powder shadow over the mistake and start again, building your color over the newly applied powder. If the mistake is more extreme and can't be corrected with powder, you might need to cover it over with foundation.

## Using Blusher

Once you have located the course of your cheekbone, putting blusher in place is relatively easy. The basic principle is to blend your rouge *under* and over the cheekbones, to bring out their shape and add definition to your face.

To put on a powder blusher, use your blush to draw a line just *under* the cheekbone, starting at the point directly beneath the outside corner of your eye and working out and up toward the tip of your ear. Continuing to work out and up in a circular motion, *blend until the line becomes a shadow* that fills in the area under the cheekbone.

For mousses and cream blushers that you apply with a sponge, the technique is much the same. But be careful not to use too much; no woman looks attractive with heavily colored cheeks. When using a sponge to apply blusher it's essential to work with a very light hand. And, especially with mousses and gels, work quickly.

## Highlighters

Once your blusher is in place you can play up the contour of the cheekbone with highlighter.

Highlighter, an eye-catching light wash of color blended *over* the cheekbone, accentuates the height of the bone, enabling it to stand out in contrast to the darker blusher color below. My favorite highlighter for daytime is my undereye concealer, which is just light enough in color to contrast nicely with my blusher. A lighter-colored rouge than the one you've put on under your cheekbone is also an excellent highlighter. Or you can use a glitter gel, or a pencil, blended in with a sponge.

# OPENING THE WINDOW TO YOUR PERSONALITY— EYE MAKEUPS

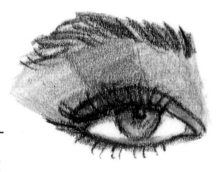
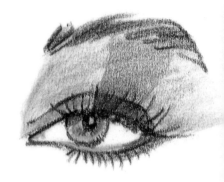

When you really look at someone—when you want to know what she feels, what she thinks, what she knows, in short, what makes her tick—you look at her eyes. Eyes speak; through them, we can communicate our innermost feelings without words; they are, indeed, the windows to our personalities.

We are indeed fortunate that we can enhance these most expressive, interesting, and individual of features. In my life at the salon, I've heard countless questions about them: How can I make my eyes bigger, brighter, lighter, darker, bluer, more mysterious, more open, more expressive, more beautiful? How can my eyes enhance my feelings of happiness; how can I hide the sadness of a broken heart? Amazingly, what we do with our lashes and brows, and how we color with shadow and pencil, profoundly affects how we are perceived, and how we see ourselves.

## Shadow

Shadow—the color you sweep on your eyelids and beneath your bottom lashes—can wake up your look, enhance and accent eye color, and express a great deal about your personality. Shadows come in a variety of forms and a cornucopia of colors; which ones you choose and how you apply them can help you to communicate your moods and your feelings as no other cosmetic can.

### Shadow Forms

**Powder shadows** are familiar to almost everyone who wears makeup because anybody can wear them. Women with oily skin find that color shadows applied over a base have great holding power. Even those with dry skin can enjoy the range of color shadows available in powder form once the skin is properly prepared with moisturizer and foundation. Best of all, a powder shadow applied over a good foundation will last all day, adding a true 9-to-5 touch of color that will not wear off as your activities wear on.

Powder shadows are extraordinarily versatile: Shadow palettes range from purse to tabletop size and hold a variety of colors, with choices limited only by your imagination and the size of your palette. They can contour, highlight, even reshape eyes. In short, they are a joy to experiment with.

**Flat matte powder shadows** are one of those fashion accessories that look right just about anytime. They can be the basis of an understated, pulled-together daytime look, and yet they can be worked into truly dazzling nightplay makeups as well. Since you can apply powder shadows with a brush rather than a sponge-tip applicator, highly subtle application and intricate shading effects are at your fingertips. All in all, I have no reservations about saying that for most people, flat matte powder shadows are one of the most truly versatile and important of all cosmetics.

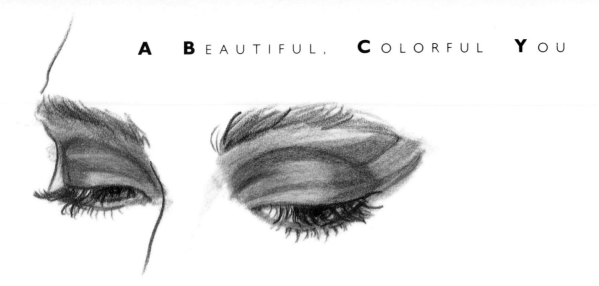

**Iridescent powder shadows,** on the other hand, are the stuff that dreams are made of. When the mood of the evening is highly charged, when the occasion sparkles, the glow of an iridescent shadow over your eye is fitting— and very flattering under artificial light. Iridescents are not for everyone, however; older women can't wear them because they accentuate the lines over the lid (flat shadows or pencils are more flattering), and they can be irritating to those with sensitive skin.

Iridescent shadows can also be effective *highlighters* for day. The sparkle of an iridescent highlighter is picked up by sunlight when used over a cream shadow; it's a lovely outdoor eye look for winter or summer.

**Cream shadows,** which are oil-based, are a boon for those whose eyes need extra moisturizing. If powders tend to be drying even over the proper base, if powder colors do not glide smoothly over your lid, opt for the emollient protection of creams when you choose your shadows. I also recommend creams for people with normal skin who are going to the beach or ski slopes, where skin tends to dry out. Or for anyone who likes a creamy finish.

**Neon cream shadows** are the eyeshadow equivalent of the popular mousse blushers. They are new, and designed for everyone. Neons come in pastel shades; what distinguishes them from other cream shadows is the "wet look" that remains even after they dry. They're fun to wear, particularly when you want a special summertime makeup look.

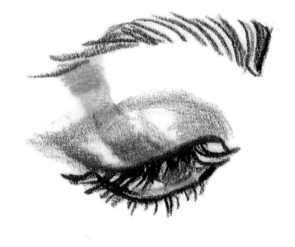

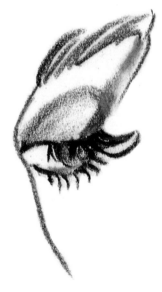

## If You Wear Glasses

**B**ecause eyeglass frames and lenses can diminish even the impact of a pair of very bright eyes, it's important for people who wear glasses to wear eye makeup. Choose your frame color and the tint of your lenses to enhance your natural coloring or the colors you like to wear. Then don't be afraid to use bold color around your eyes; adding complementary eye makeups will bring out the expressiveness of your eyes—it will keep you from being hidden behind your glasses.

## Pencil Looks

Pencils are extraordinary, both because they're so easy to use and because they are so versatile. A creamy eye pencil can perform a staggering variety of tasks: It can line, shape, accent, and shadow. Using one pencil, which you can carry with you wherever you go, you can create a whole makeup almost instantly.

The simplest pencil look is a line of black or brown pencil around the eyes, to define and shape them. But you needn't just outline; make a color statement as well by choosing a bright pencil shade that will bring out the clarity of your eyes.

Using a kohl pencil is another alternative. Kohl is a makeup that has been used for centuries in India and the Middle East. It's a natural cosmetic, a charcoal-colored sand, and it's very soft. It's a beautiful cosmetic to work with both for its interesting, smoky texture and for its hypoallergenic qualities, which make it much easier on sensitive eyes than ordinary pencils.

Since kohl pencils are both very soft and hypoallergenic, they are perfectly formulated for use along the rim inside your lashes. (But make sure your pencil says "kohl" before you use it there.) Kohl can be used as a conventional liner along the lashes as well, but because it's so soft, it tends to smear. I prefer using it on the inside only. Draw a line of kohl inside your lashes and your eyes will look brighter in seconds.

When you use kohl without a shadow or pencil around the outside of the rim, it can have a narrowing effect. Widen your eye by using a shadow or drawing a line of pencil around the lashes.

## Opening Your Eyes

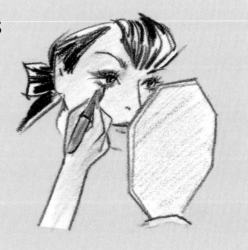

**A** line of pencil drawn *under* the bottom lashes and the outer corner of your eye has an eye-opening effect. Blend shadow over the pencil for a more colorful eye-opener.

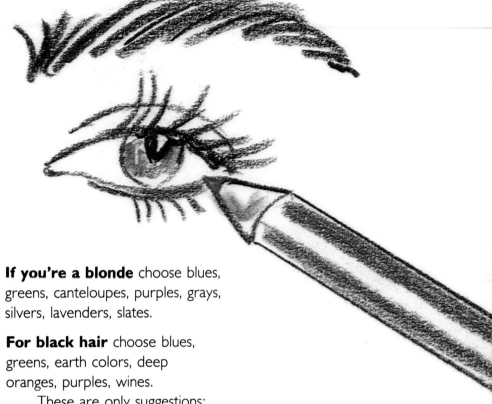

## Pencil Colors

Black or very dark brown pencils almost shout "dramatic." Anyone can wear these dark shades, but for them to be effective you must go all the way and team them with equally dramatic dark blue or charcoal shadows. If you want a light, pretty effect, dark pencils will overshadow and detract from your look.

For daytime wear, I'd suggest shades that are a little lighter and more colorful than blacks and dark browns. Keeping in mind that your eye pencil should be slightly more emphatic than your shadow color, team pencils with matching or contrasting shadows. The following shades will enhance your eye color as well as your makeup look:

**For red hair** choose blues, greens, turquoises, golds.

**If you have dark hair/brown eyes** choose blues, greens, purples, lavenders, maroons, golds.

**If you're a blonde** choose blues, greens, canteloupes, purples, grays, silvers, lavenders, slates.

**For black hair** choose blues, greens, earth colors, deep oranges, purples, wines.

These are only suggestions; you can break your personal color barrier with as few or as many pencil colors as you keep in your makeup kit.

## Applying Shadow and Pencil Color

First things first: Before you apply your shadow and pencil, blend in concealer where you need it and be sure to remember your lids and below your bottom lashes when you're putting on your foundation. And when you dust with transparent powder, dust over your eyes as well as the rest of your face. Your shadow will last as long as your day does.

SHADOW TECHNIQUES
A small brush, preferably the type known as a fluff brush, is essential in applying powder shadows to your lid, and a small, wedge-shaped brush is most effective under your bottom lashes.

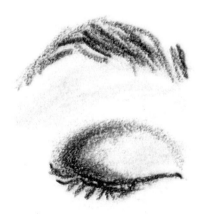

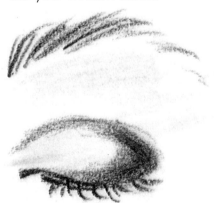

Your brushes allow you to apply shadow color a stroke at a time and to blend lines of color into true shadows. So put aside the sponge-tip applicator that came with your shadow palette; your brushes will give you a far subtler and smoother finish. They will also enable you to blend color into color, building an eye makeup out of several different shadow shades. Blend each straight line of shadow into the next, eliminating as you go any lines that have a separate appearance.

If you are using iridescent powder shadows, however, a sponge-tip applicator will hold the iridescent pigment much better than a brush and is preferable.

If you want to create an eye-liner look with your cream shadows, use a flat, thin brush for application.

BLENDING SHADOWS

For a complete makeup, you will probably be blending several different shadows together. Start by applying an ivory powder shadow as a base; it will absorb moisture and even out the skin color of your lids. Blend it in well with your brush before adding other shadows. Next you might choose to apply a contour shadow under your bottom lashes and in the crease of the eye. Remember, your relatively dark contour shade will cause those potentially puffy

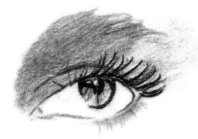

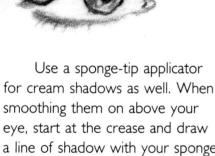

## If Your Shadow Disappears into the Crease of Your Eye

**W**hether you're using powder or cream shadows, you need to prime your lids to prevent disappearing shadows. Be sure to blend your foundation onto your eyelids, and always follow with transparent powder. Then prime with an ivory powder shadow. Stroke the primer on with a medium-sized flat brush before putting on your color shadows.

Use a sponge-tip applicator for cream shadows as well. When smoothing them on above your eye, start at the crease and draw a line of shadow with your sponge tip. Blend up or down from the crease, depending on the effect you want from the shadow.

areas to recede in relation to lighter-shaded surroundings. Apply a lighter color shadow on the lower part of your lid and add a light highlighter right below your eyebrows. When they're blended in well with your brush (or sponge-tip applicator if you are using cream or iridescent shadows), you won't be able to tell where one shadow begins and the next leaves off.

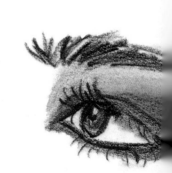

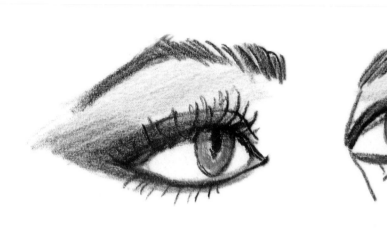

## Pencil as Accent

Create more drama by shading the outer corner of your eye with pencil. A dark blueberry or a light brown or silver shade makes a very pretty accent. And don't be afraid to experiment by accenting the inner rather than the outer corner of the lid. It creates a very interesting eye look, as you can see.

### PENCIL TECHNIQUES

The secret to outlining the eye is to keep the pencil as close as possible to the lashes. When lining under the bottom lashes, hold your pencil at an upward angle and move it back and forth with short strokes right under the lashes. When lining above your

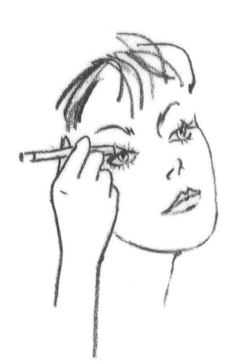

To line the inner rim of your eye with a soft-textured kohl pencil, look down and gently pull the bottom lashes away from your eye. Place the pencil inside the rim of the eye and carefully line, keeping the pencil just inside the lash line.

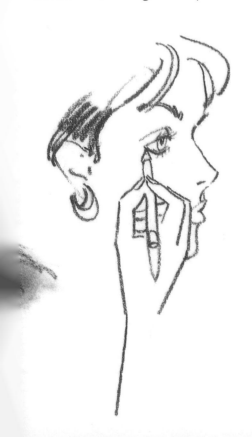

top lashes, half-close your eye to give yourself access to the space right over the lashes; hold your pencil at a downward angle and draw your line from the inside corner of your eye out.

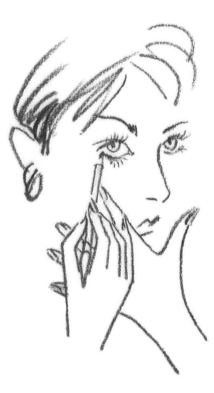

## How to Stop Your Pencil from Running

**P**encils are really a form of cream shadow. They're easy to apply because they're very soft, but some are so soft that they melt or run after you put them on. Kohl pencils are even softer; applied outside the lashes they also tend to run.

The way to stop pencils from streaking is to first apply a contour powder shadow all around your eye in a color close to that of the pencil or in a neutral shade. The powder shadow will act as a base and keep your creamy pencil from running. After drawing in your pencil line, blend it into the shadow with the thin side of your sponge-tip applicator.

black eyeliner and red lips. In our own day, we need only think of Sophia Loren to visualize her unusually long, strong eyes—accented and made dramatic by eyeliner. And who can imagine Elizabeth Taylor without the liner that focuses attention on her trademark violet eyes?

A simple line of eyeliner gives your eye a definition it can get from no other makeup. If you are looking for a pretty, understated look, use a soft-colored pencil—but for nighttime, for special effects, bold eyeliner is marvelous.

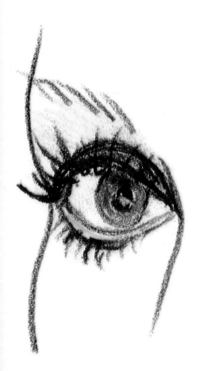

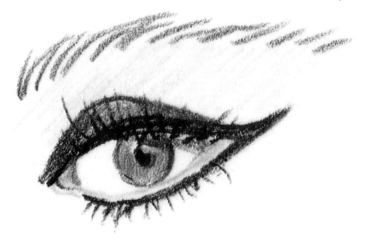

Modern-day eyeliner comes in various forms.

There is convenient, ready-to-use **liquid liner,** which comes in a small bottle with its own little brush (much like mascara).

A **pencil liner** is convenient and easy to use, but it gives you a much thicker line and the least control of application of any eyeliner form.

## For Dramatic Effect—Eyeliner

The one cosmetic that will really draw attention to your eyes is eyeliner. By lining the frames and surrounding the eyes, eyeliner shapes mood. In fact, it's been heightening the dramatic effect of

beautiful eyes for thousands of years, since the time of Cleopatra. During the heyday of Hollywood, from Harlow to Monroe, when makeups were not as colorful as they are now, the basic look was

**40**

**Cake liner,** on the other hand, gives you the most control of application. To use it, wet your eyeliner brush, dip it in the cake, and apply around your eye. With cake liner you can readily control the amount of eyeliner you use, as well as how thick or thin you draw your line.

Another alternative is **shadow liner** (using powder shadow in place of cake liner). Applied with a wedge-cut brush, shadow liner frees you from the usual eyeliner color constraints of blacks and browns; you can have any color liner you wish. The color will be more intense the shorter you cut the hairs of your brush.

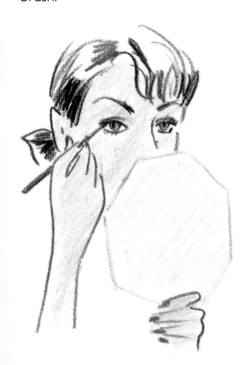

## Lash Looks

I'm a fan of the eyelash curler, a little tool that's easy to use and vastly underappreciated. I love it because it's literally an eye-opener. You can look through dozens of advertisements for mascaras and never realize that all those spectacularly curly lashes owe more to the eyelash curler than to the mascara applicator. I think it's time the eyelash curler got the appreciation it deserves as an essential to pretty and natural-looking eye makeups.

An eyelash curler looks a bit like a surgical tool, but it's actually very safe and simple to use. Take time to align your lashes between the clamps of the curler. Before you exert any pressure, make sure you've caught your lash *midway* (and be sure your bottom lashes are free). Once you've caught the lashes at midpoint, clamp firmly for about thirty seconds, then release. Your lashes will be curled, and your eye will appear larger and more open.

If you curl your lashes, there will probably be times you decide not to use mascara. But if you do use mascara, it will roll up your lashes with an ease you never thought possible. Mascara brushes were made for curled lashes.

## Mascara and Color

Charcoal, black, and dark brown are the basic, conservative shades of mascara. I would choose an outright black only if I wanted to make a really dramatic statement, and then I'd team it with a charcoal or dark gray shadow or a line of black outlining pencil or eyeliner. In general, I find that colored mascaras are much more effective as a finishing touch for a light, fresh makeup look than conventional dark shades are. I personally use brown or dark brown mascaras as basic shades because of my brown eyes and hair. If I had black hair I'd opt for a blue-black mascara rather than straight black as a basic shade. If I had auburn hair I'd choose a wine color, and if I were a blonde I'd consider blues or greens as basic shades.

The first time someone sees you in a colored mascara they'll tell you one of two things: how pretty you look, or, if they're a little more perceptive, how fresh you look. Because the lovely thing about colored mascaras is that they *are* fresh-looking.

## Special Effects Mascara

**C**ombine a black and a colored mascara for a devastating special effect. Apply your black mascara to the base of your lashes for drama. Then "tip" your lashes with a colored mascara that enhances the tones of your shadows. The effect is really different—and fabulous.

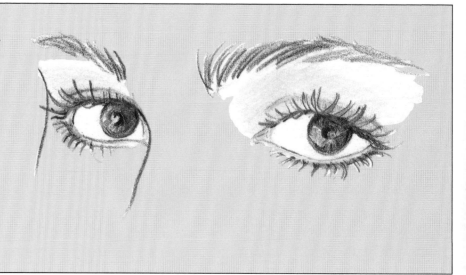

Colored mascara looks its best when it matches your eye pencil—for instance, blue on blue or wine on wine. You can also co-ordinate your shadows and mascaras so that you have brighter blue mascaras with slightly darker blue shadows, or green-brown mascaras with yellow-brown shadows. Or you can play up the color of your mascara by teaming it with a different-colored shadow, as I do when I put a violet mascara with a pink or blue shadow, a wine mascara with a brown shadow, or a pink shadow with a blue mascara and blue pencil. So you can see that blues and pinks are not just for blondes.

## For Blonde Lashes

**I**f you have blonde or light lashes and your skin is not sensitive, tinting gives you the option of going without mascara for your daytime makeups. Done by a professional in a salon, eyelash tinting is a very simple procedure that lasts four to six weeks. Because no harsh chemicals are used—it's done with a harmless vegetable dye (I use a henna dye at *il Makiage*)—there is no danger of irritation to normal skin. And it works beautifully. Imagine waking up with the kind of dark, well-defined eyes other women must take the time to put on.

When you have your lashes tinted, ask for a dye that isn't too dark, maybe a dark brown for a light look or a blue-black for a darker look. You can always add mascara later for a dramatic long-lash effect.

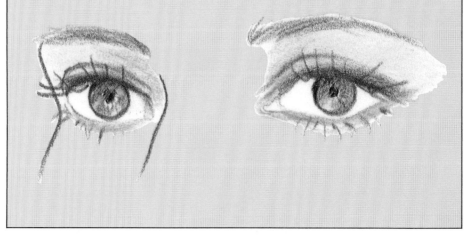

## Applying Mascara

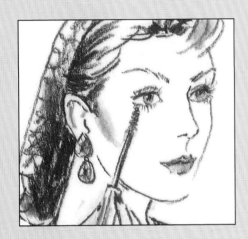

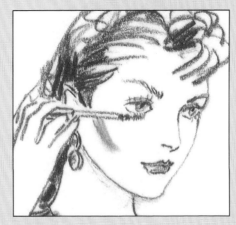

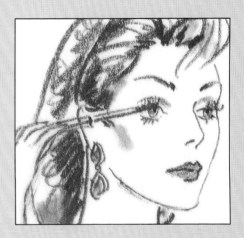

**1.** *Begin with your bottom lashes.* If you start at the top you could get little splatter marks all over your eyelid when you look up to begin the bottom lashes.

**2.** When you apply mascara under the bottom lashes, first move the tip of your wand back and forth over the lashes to apply color. Then place the wand under the lashes and roll it up and out to distribute color and separate the lashes.

**3.** Begin to color your upper lashes from the top side and roll your mascara wand gently up the curl of the lashes before stroking the ends. Allow a few seconds for the mascara to dry.

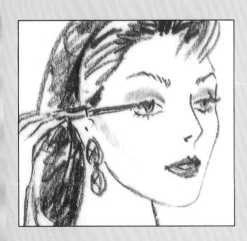

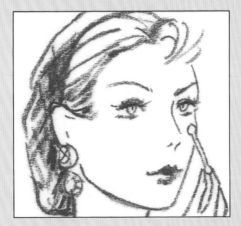

**4.** Next, roll your wand up the inside of the lashes so that you exaggerate the curl as well as coat the lashes. Again, stroke the ends.

**5.** Resist the temptation to scrub at a smudge with tissue. Instead, put a cotton swab up against the splatter mark and twist it slightly so that the mascara comes away on the cotton tip.

# SHAPE YOUR PERSONALITY— EYEBROWS

*Eyebrows define a character.* In 1925, before she became a star, Joan Crawford's eyebrows were almost straight across, just slightly downturned. Her face—and her character—became etched in our memories only when she changed her eyebrows to that dark, arched look she made famous. We re-member the inquisitive, round, high brows of Marlene Deitrich, the narrow arches of Elizabeth Taylor's brows, the brushed-up brows of Sophia Loren. In the late 1970's, Margaux Hemingway and then Brooke Shields created a new fashion; their brushed-up but essentially untouched, natural-looking brows have replaced the narrow, arched look of the 1950's and 1960's.

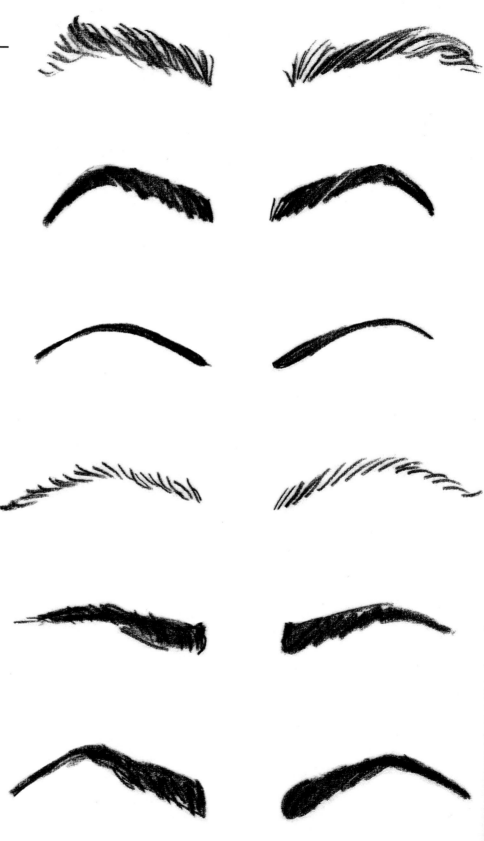

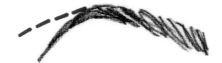 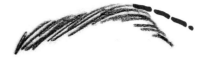

Your brows are a combination of what nature has given you and how your personality defines your nature. There are no hard-and-fast rules as far as eyebrow shaping is concerned, and you need not change your own inquisitive-looking brows despite the heavier-looking brows all around you. Generally, I prefer lighter-looking brows for day and stronger, more "lifted" brows for evening. And I also think people look better with more arched eyebrows as they get older. The slight sag that occurs just over the eye and under the brow is visually reduced by taking away hairs to lift the brows. And lifting the eyebrows has almost the effect of a mini-facelift; it can make you look ten years younger.

## How to Shape Your Eyebrows

Imagine a straight line going up from the outside of your nostril through the inner corner of your eye; that line defines where your brow should begin. Now imagine a line going from the outside of your nostril past the outer corner of your eye; that's where your brow should

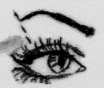

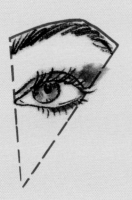

end. You can tweeze away hairs that exceed these boundaries or extend brows with a pencil line to reach them.

Another general brow-shaping guideline is to take excess hairs away from below the arch of the brow rather than above it. This not only lifts the eye visually, it keeps the natural arch of the brow intact. Only take off hair from the top if you have dark, thick hair (in which case waxing is advisable); otherwise, removing more than a hair or two from the top of your brows will tend to flatten your look.

## Color and Shape with Eyebrow Pencil

Lighter, distinctively arched brows begin when you use pencil. Pencil is also the easiest way, short of bleaching or tinting, to put color into brows that are colorless or the wrong color.

An auburn is very useful for anyone with hair that has reddish highlights, because the auburn will mask the gray that sometimes steals into your brows. If you have chestnut-brown hair, a gray-brown pencil is a good basic shade; if you have honey-colored hair, try a light brown. I like a taupe for fair brows and a charcoal for dark brows. (Black is strictly for the special effects Crawford look.) And if you have recently become a platinum blonde, one way to deal with leftover eyebrows is to put on a gray pencil when you're wearing black or gray clothes, and a taupe pencil when you're wearing browns or beiges. And if you want a special nighttime charcoal look, try a silver eyebrow pencil.

Before you pencil your brows, brush them. This will clarify their natural shape and also allow you to focus on any thin or uneven spots. Then, holding your

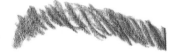

pencil at an angle so that you can get between the hairs easily, fill in your brow with short, feathery strokes of color.

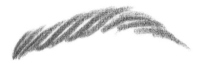

## Eyebrow Color

**U**nless you are a genuine blonde with naturally darker brows, your eyebrows should be the same shade as, or a shade lighter than, your hair. It's a nuisance to have to mask eyebrow color day after day; a few minutes can take care of it for weeks at a time. If your eyebrow color is way off you can have your eyebrows tinted or bleached at your salon. A good time to do it is when you henna, color, or bleach your hair, because that's when many of us end up with brows that don't match. But do consult with a professional first. This is not a procedure for women with sensitive skin. Nor should it be done at home.

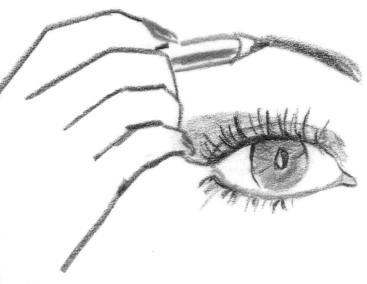

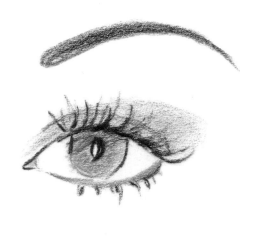

## Eyebrow Set

These days, most of us keep our brows fairly natural looking. Brooke Shields was among the first to popularize this natural look, capitalizing on her wide-open eyes and brushed-up brows. Brooke's secret for maintaining her look is eyebrow set. It's the softest, simplest, sweetest way to treat natural-looking brows.

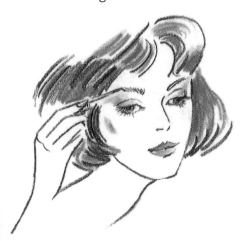

Eyebrow set comes in a bottle with an applicator brush, so it's very easy to use. It's clear, like gloss, and it helps brows stay in place for hours. Once you've brushed your brows up, stroke on your eyebrow set; it will give your brows a slight shine and give you a bright, open-eyed look.

## Mascara for a Special Effect

Now that you've broken the color barrier, it's time to break the usage barrier as well. Many cosmetics, like pencils, rouges, even eye color, can do double-duty. Mascara might sound out of place as an eyebrow cosmetic, but the product you use to dramatize your lashes can rev up your brows as well. Mascara, unlike eyebrow set, actually stiffens the brows to help them stay where you want them—brush them up and you'll achieve a special, high-impact nighttime look.

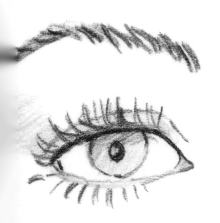

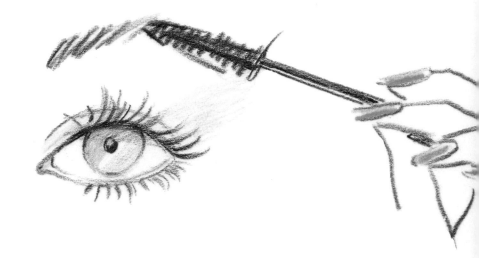

# COLOR AND SHAPE YOUR MOOD— LIP MAKEUPS

Lips are in many ways as expressive as eyes. Smiling or pouting, boldly or subtly colored, simply or irresistibly shaped—*your lips and the makeups you wear on them are great communicators of mood.*

Recently, at a photo session for this book, I had the opportunity to observe and make up the well-known model Debbie Dickinson, who has the most amazing, expressive lips: Every time her mood changes, the very shape of her lips seems to go through a metamorphosis as well. Debbie's lips are a wonderful beauty asset (and she *is* one of a kind), but anyone's lips can be made more beautiful, more sensual, and more exciting if she's willing to break the color barrier.

## Choosing Your Lipstick—Stay Out of the Color Trap

Even people who are adventurous about the clothes they wear often get trapped by the same old lip colors. It's almost as if they've forgotten that their lips are part of them and that their lip makeup is an essential part of their total look. The other day, for example,

a very attractive dark-haired, dark-eyed woman came into the salon wearing a striking deep maroon jacket—and bright red lipstick. I easily pulled her look together with a brown lip shade. Not only did the earthy tone complement the color of her jacket, but it brought out the luster in her hair and eyes.

*Match your lip makeup to your clothes*: It's one of my favorite strategies for breaking the color barrier. You've got a virtual rainbow of choices, from reds to peaches to pinks to browns to oranges to purples to lavenders. Start with your basic colors, but I guarantee that soon you'll be wearing lipstick shades you never thought possible.

## Lip Moods

**Soft.** Gloss gives you an easy daytime look with a subtle, soft glow. When you choose shades that match your predominant lip color (such as a pink gloss over pinkish-colored lips or a cherry gloss over cherry-toned lips), the sheen of the gloss will emphasize the natural look of your lips in a very simple, pretty way.

**Impressive.** *Lipstick provides a touch of authority that can't be matched by a gloss,* since even a pale shade of lipstick has more intense color than any gloss. Choose a lipstick if your makeup mood calls for something simple, classic, and eye-catching. And even if you usually use gloss, try a

lipstick the next time you have an important daytime occasion; it will make a difference.

**Seductive.** For a sexier, more seductive look, try combining the shininess of a gloss and the color of a lipstick in one makeup. For maximum color, put a matching shade of gloss over your lipstick, rather than using a transparent gloss.

**Smashing.** For something really special, consider this: After outlining your lips with pencil, fill in the top lip and the corners of the bottom lip with a bold lipstick shade, then slick a lighter shade of gloss across the center of the lower lip. Your mouth will appear fuller, more rounded, absolutely lush. And if you're in the mood for an eye-catching makeup that's a little softer looking, use a lighter shade of lipstick instead of the light gloss.

## Creating Beautiful Lips

Every woman has many makeup moods. There are occasions when you simply won't have the time or the inclination to create an elaborate makeup. And there are times when you'll do everything you can to enhance and dramatize your natural beauty. But whatever your makeup mood, there are no shortcuts to truly long-lasting lips.

## Special Tips for Luscious Lips

### IF YOUR LIPSTICK COMES OFF ON YOUR GLASS

Creamier-textured lipsticks often seem to come off on everything they touch, while lipsticks that have a fairly dry texture have more staying power. How can you tell which is which? The drier-textured lipsticks contain more pigmentation, which means that the redder your lipstick, the more likely it is to stay on. (Lipsticks that contain iridescent pigment are also long-lasting.) If you favor the creamier-textured, more muted lipsticks, try blotting your lips gently with a tissue before sitting down to a meal at your favorite restaurant. Excess lipstick will come off on the tissue, not on your glass, but you will have enough color left on your lips so you'll still look as if you have a full makeup.

### IF YOUR LIPSTICK CHANGES COLOR ON YOUR LIPS

Your lips probably have a blue undertone to them that shows through lipstick and lip gloss colors. This is quite common, particularly among people with relatively sallow skin. Try priming with a white lipstick to cover up the undertone before you put on your colors.

### WHITE LIPSTICK FOR A DEEP TAN

If you are planning a sun-filled summer, keep this in mind: White lipstick is extraordinarily effective when used alone over lips that contrast with deeply tanned skin.

### DRY LIPS

If you smoke or drink a lot of coffee, if you ski or sail, if you wear iridescent or long-lasting lipsticks, or if you just want to prevent uncomfortable lip dryness, lip balm is indispensable. It moisturizes and helps prevent chapped lips and cold sores. In fact, there are so many good reasons to use lip balm I can't think of a single reason not to. And if you have very full lips or want a no-makeup/makeup look, you might even want to use it alone to give your lips a shiny, and protective, finish.

## Preparing Your Lips for Color

One persistent problem that many women have with lip color is that their lipstick "bleeds" off into the fine lines of skin around their lips. It's very easy to do away with this problem once and for all.

When you put foundation on your face in the morning, blend it right into your lips as well. If you are using lip balm as a lip moisturizer, put it on right on top of your foundation. And if your mood calls for your lips to stand out, follow by drawing a line of concealer all around your lips. The lighter color will focus all the attention where you want it. Once you've brushed your lips with transparent powder, they will be ready for color. Your lip line will not "bleed," and your gloss or lipstick will stay bright. And the whole process takes hardly more time than it took to read about it.

## Outlining Your Lips

Outlining gives lip makeup a finished look as well as further protecting your lipsticks and glosses from smudging and bleeding. And *outlining makes your lips more beautiful* by emphasizing their shape so that they appear fuller, rounder, and more desirable.

Outlining requires a small brush or an outlining pencil. Brushes produce a more meticulous result; pencils are faster and easier to use.

Lips are very sensitive; use only soft-textured, well-sharpened pencils on them. You can select pencil shades to match your lip-sticks or glosses, or you can choose slightly darker pencils. Remember, dark recedes, light emphasizes; the darker line around the lips will thrust your lighter-colored lipstick or gloss into greater prominence, thus accentuating your lips' fullness.

Outlining is relatively simple when you use the following method. Before attempting to draw in a full outline, put one dot at each peak of your Cupid's bow; follow each dot straight down to the bottom of your lower lip and draw in two more dots. Connect both upper and lower lip dots in the center and then draw each line out to the end of your lips.

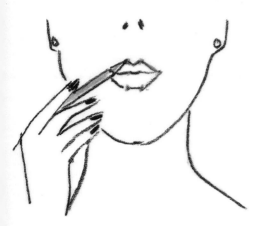

**Applying Lipstick or Gloss**

Lip color, straight from the tube, seems convenient and easy to use. However, most women are unable to trace the lip lines with a thick, unwieldy lipstick. There is a better way. A tube of lip color that is applied with its own sponge-tip applicator or a sable lip brush used with lipstick will give you a more even application and longer-lasting lip color.

## Your Gloss Is Too Sheer to Cover Your Outlining Pencil

**U**sing lip pencil with a transparent gloss can be a problem. I "erase" leftover pencil lines with a technique I call lip tinting. After you have outlined your lips and applied your gloss, simply take your lip brush and blend the lip liner into the gloss. It will give you a shiny, translucent, subtle-looking finish.

Another alternative is to blend your pencil all over your lips to give you a stain and dispense with gloss completely.

Dip your brush tip into your lipstick or gloss and then stroke the color onto your lips. The brush will give you enough control to blend your lipstick all the way into your lip outline, thus softening the sharpness of the line into a smoothly blended and colored whole.

Because of the fabulously improved results you'll get with a lip brush, after using it just a few times I doubt you'll ever again be tempted to use lipstick straight from the tube.

If you want the more dramatic look of lip gloss over lipstick or two lipstick shades in one makeup, blend the different colors together with your brush so that there is no clear line where one leaves off and the other begins.

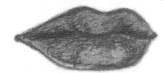

**Shaping Your Lips**

Whether you love the shape of your lips or want to compensate for nature's shortcomings, you can

have fun reshaping your lips whenever the mood strikes. You can give yourself rounder, fuller lips or lips that are more demure. But lip shaping isn't merely a question of making your lips larger or smaller; using that amazing little tool, your outlining pencil, you can create a wide variety of lip shapes (and moods) easily. You will find that one or two small touches can change your entire appearance.

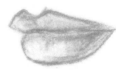

**To subtly exaggerate lip size,** use your lip pencil to draw a line slightly outside the natural line of your lips. Fill in the new shape with your color and brush, making sure that you blend in the pencil line with your lipstick or gloss.

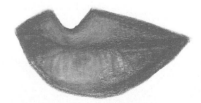

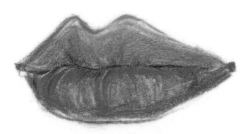

**If your mood calls for smaller lips,** exactly the same technique applies except that you draw your pencil line *inside* the natural line of your lips.

## New Lip Shapes Over Old

With lip shaping you can even put one makeup mood over another. For example, at eight this morning you left your house with a simple lip look of gloss over your naturally outlined lip line. Now evening approaches, and you want to make your lips look fuller and sexier. You don't even have to remove your original lip makeup. Here's what you do: First blot out your old lip shape by reapplying foundation, drawing a new line of concealer, and then repowdering your lips. Follow by penciling in a new outline and adding color.

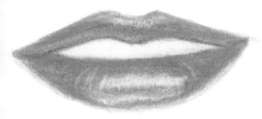

**To emphasize your new lip shape,** draw a line of white outlining pencil outside the line of your regular-colored pencil.

## The Effect of Color on Lip Shape

The type and intensity of color you use on your lips has a big effect on their apparent shape.

Gloss will make a narrow mouth appear wider.

Use very little lipstick on narrow lips; using a lot just accentuates your natural lip shape.

Bright colors make big lips appear even bigger. Use a clear gloss or a soft-colored lipstick instead.

Using a gloss only in the center of your lips will plump your mouth and also prevent your gloss from running.

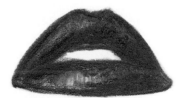

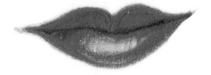

**To make rounder-looking lips,** draw your pencil line slightly outside the natural lip line as you turn the corners of your mouth. Once you've filled in your lips with lipstick (blending, always blending), blot the corners softly with a tissue to further mute the rounded pencil line into a natural look.

**To "lift" unhappy-looking lips** that turn down slightly at the corners, draw the bottom lip line slightly up and out at the corners. Pencil in the upper corners to meet the new line of your lower lip.

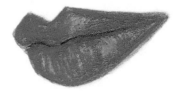

# FOR A FINISHING TOUCH— COLORED POWDER

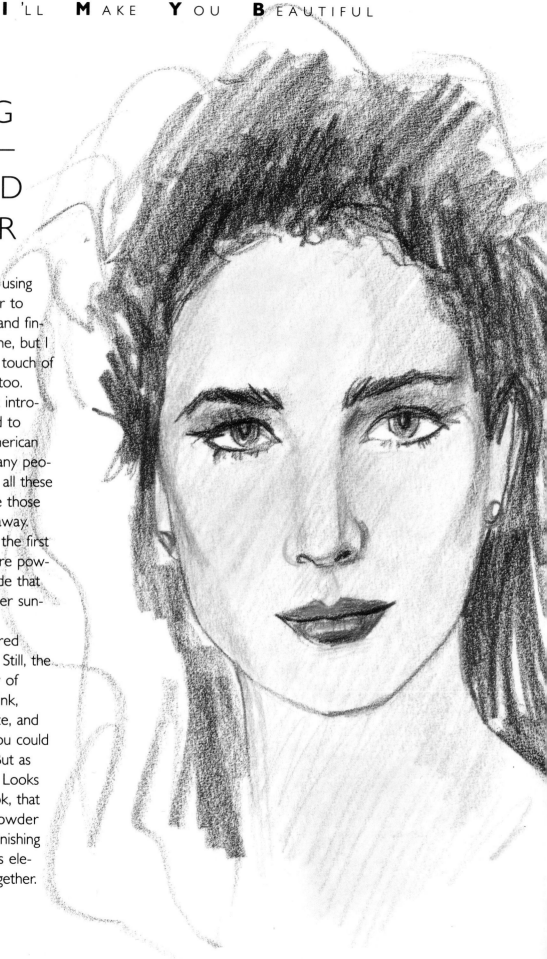

You are probably used to using the same shade of powder to both set your foundation and finish your makeup. That's fine, but I often like to add an extra touch of color, and I think you will too.

When *il-Makiage* first introduced colored as opposed to tinted powders to the American public a few years ago, many people wondered—what are all these colors for? But there were those who took to them right away. Raquel Welch was among the first to use one of my adventure powders, a yellow-bronze shade that perfectly complemented her suntanned California look.

Now, of course, colored powders are everywhere. Still, the first time you see an array of powder colors including pink, peach, coral, yellow, bronze, and violet you may feel that you could never wear such shades. But as you will see in "The Many Looks of You," Part 2 of this book, that final dusting of colored powder can well be the beautiful finishing touch that pulls the various elements of your makeup together.

How can you begin to use colored powders confidently? Pinks, peaches, tans, and bronzes are the easiest to start with because, at first sight, they don't appear as outrageous as some of the other "special effects" colors.

If you are a blonde or a brunette with fair skin, plan a makeup around pink or peach blusher, shadows, and gloss. Once your blusher, shadow, and lip gloss are all in place, lightly dust with a pink or peach powder to finish the look.

Tans and bronze shades of colored powder are excellent for people who have brown hair and skin that is beige or darker than beige. They will give your skin a warm look. If you are in a holiday mood, simply pull out a bronze-tinted powder and give yourself an instant tan by whisking the powder across your face and over your nose and cheeks. In two seconds you'll look as if you spent the week outdoors rather than in the office.

The best way to use special effects shades like violet or yellow is to do what Raquel Welch did with her colored powders: Match them with eyeshadows and pencils to give your makeup a unified color theme. It's a makeup idea that works beautifully when you're in a sophisticated mood.

## Using Colored Powder as the Basis of a Quick Makeup Look

Colored powder can create a lovely, transparent makeup look almost all by itself. Use colored powder in contour areas or as a sheer shadow and blusher all in one to give a touch of color to a pale face. With the addition of lipstick or gloss, you've created a fabulous minimal makeup look.

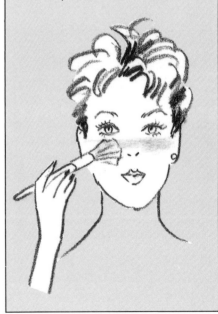

# QUICK-AS-A-WINK MAKEUP LOOKS

Every woman knows the situation: an important meeting, a sudden, impetuous date, a clock that never stops insisting you're late for work. Whatever the specifics, the result is that you have little or no time to put on your makeup. What do you do? Do you give up? Do you bury your head and go back to bed? Do you delude yourself into thinking it doesn't matter how you look? Or do you run around like a crazy person, slapping whatever is at hand onto your face? Is looking good an impossible dream?

If you start your day with a coffee cup in one hand and an eye pencil in the other, with one eye on the clock and the other on the door, it may seem like there's no solution—but there is.

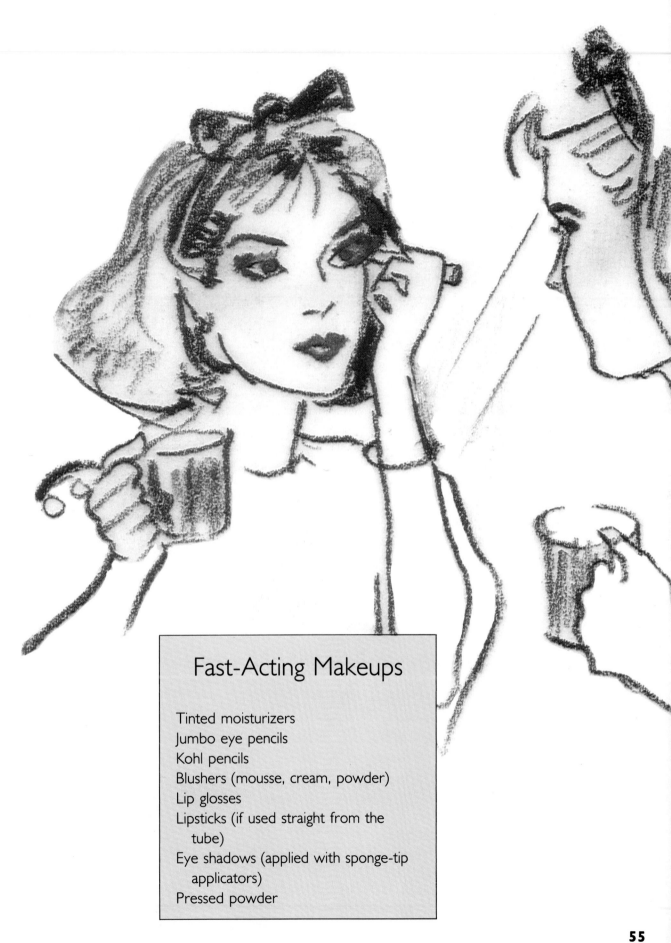

## Fast-Acting Makeups

Tinted moisturizers
Jumbo eye pencils
Kohl pencils
Blushers (mousse, cream, powder)
Lip glosses
Lipsticks (if used straight from the
    tube)
Eye shadows (applied with sponge-tip
    applicators)
Pressed powder

# FIVE MINUTES TO GO

Make up and be ready to go in five minutes or less? Why not?

*The essence of a fast makeup is simplicity*, and simplicity is the basis for a long-lasting, beautifully finished daytime look. To get out the door and on your way in minutes, you'll have to rethink your makeup strategies. You can't possibly put together a state-of-the-art nighttime makeup look in less than five minutes, but you *can* create a lasting, polished effect. And you can achieve that colorful pulled-together look using only a handful of cosmetics.

So how do you bring out your best if you only have five minutes to go? Take a few minutes now to formulate a streamlined plan and you'll be on your way before you know it.

## Essential Ingredients

| MAKEUPS | TOOLS |
|---|---|
| Moisturizer | Makeup sponges |
| Concealer | Cotton swabs |
| Foundation or pressed powder | |
| Loose transparent powder | Powder brush |
| Mousse or powder blusher | Blusher brush |
| Cream or powder shadow | Sponge-tip applicator or fluff brush |
| Eye pencil | Eyelash curler |
| Lip pencil | Lip brush |
| Matching lip gloss or lipstick | Tissues, etc. |

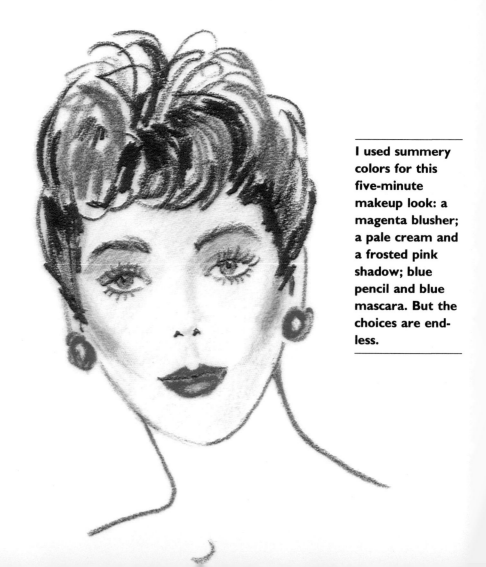

**I used summery colors for this five-minute makeup look: a magenta blusher; a pale cream and a frosted pink shadow; blue pencil and blue mascara. But the choices are endless.**

# WAKE UP TO COLOR

Color is the key to a fast, fresh look. If you use color inventively, you can rely on the same basic makeup techniques morning after morning and still come up with a lively makeup every day.

A makeup that's composed entirely of neutral shades makes you look older and tired—so wake up to color; it'll put you in a good mood even when you're tired or overworked. You may only have time for a little lipstick, a pencil, or an eyeshadow, but that's enough time to make a difference. Color brings out those features people see first—your eyes and lips—so why look dowdy because you have an early morning meeting? A fresh, well-groomed look, a little color over lips and eyes—that's all you need for the perfect quick-as-a-wink daytime makeup.

Cold colors and warm colors work equally well for a daytime look, so consider your mood before you pull out your makeups. If you're expecting a hard day, go with warmer colors; they will add a little warmth to your face and take some of the chill off even the longest business meeting. But remember, even some pinks can be quite cold looking unless you have a naturally warm skin tone.

---

## Double-Duty Cosmetics

**M**ousse and powder blushers, which double as lipsticks and shadows

**E**ye pencils, which can be used as highlighters, rouges, and lip pencils

**F**lat matte powder shadows, which can double as almost anything

---

If you find you're getting caught in a color trap, wearing the same one or two colors day after day, reach for lavenders instead of blues, melons instead of browns. Or if you always wear darker shades, try pastels. A blond, blue-eyed friend of mine once complained that everyone always put her in dark pencils and shadows ("everyone" being typical cosmetics counter salespeople); I gave her a different look by suggesting a pinkish-red for eyeshadow and lip gloss, thus avoiding the opposite color cliché, those "pink" pinks that used to be ubiquitous on blondes. As for people who normally favor pastels, I'd start with one dark shadow as an accent in the outer corner of the eye, to get used to the look of darker shades.

Color choice is particularly important when you spend your day under fluorescent lights. Fluorescents wash away color; they make you look pale, even sallow, as though you have less makeup on than you actually do. If your color seems washed out, check your foundation shade. Or you could need a lavender-shaded toner to counteract the yellow tones of the lighting. But to overcome the cast of fluorescent lighting once and for all, choose shades that give color to your skin—warm-looking browns, blues, pinks, eggplants.

A different color strategy applies if you're spending your day in natural light. Color is intensified by sunlight, so any little bit of color you apply will look much more colorful once you step outdoors.

# FAST-ACTING AND DOUBLE-DUTY COSMETICS

When you're pressed for time, reach for a cosmetic that will go on in seconds and doesn't require every ounce of your concentration. Rely on a jumbo eye pencil, for example, rather than an eyeliner and brush.

Experiment with cosmetics that will do double duty for your look. If you brush powder or cream blusher over your lips and eyes as well as your cheeks, you won't have to rummage through your makeup kit to come up with matching shades of lipstick and eyeshadow.

# FIVE MINUTES TO A LONG-LASTING LOOK

Apply moisturizer in a three-dot pattern, *but use it only where you need it*. If you have oily skin or an oily T-zone, clean oily areas with astringent lotion.

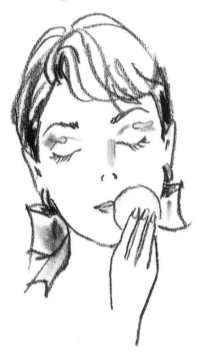

Squeeze a few drops of foundation onto a corner of your folded makeup sponge and blend your foundation where you most need the coverage. Dab a loose powder that matches your foundation over your face, concentrating primarily on the T-zone area. That's where oiliness is most likely to break through first.

Next, use a flexible makeup sponge to apply your mousse blusher. (I've chosen a mousse and sponge for this makeup, but a powder rouge and brush work equally well.) Place three dots of mousse blusher in a line parallel to (and under) each cheekbone. Gently blend with your sponge, working out and up (but always under the cheekbone) until the three dots have turned into a shadow. Refold your sponge whenever you think you've picked up too much blusher, or you won't get the transparent finish you want. Once you've finished with your cheeks, blend leftover rouge into the hairline and around the jawline to give you a little more color. Blend in a touch of concealer over the cheekbones as a natural-looking highlighter.

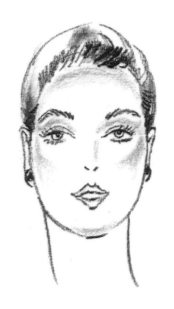

Cream shadows (including neon cream shadows), applied with a sponge-tip applicator, go on faster than powder shadows. And they can be applied directly over moisturizer. To speed up the application of a powder shadow, use a sponge-tip applicator instead of a brush. And always start with a neutral-colored shadow base over your lid; this will ensure that your color shadows go on smoothly— and stay on.

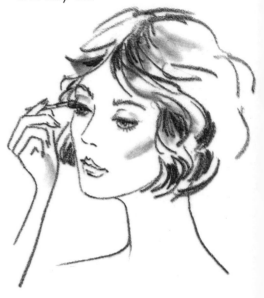

Smooth a line of shadow along the crease of the eye, then blend up with the broad tip of your applicator until the line has become a shadow. You can fill in the area under the browbone or leave room for a highlighter, which can be a neutral shade of concealer or a lighter-colored shadow. Sweep a soft, lighter shade across the lower part of your lid.

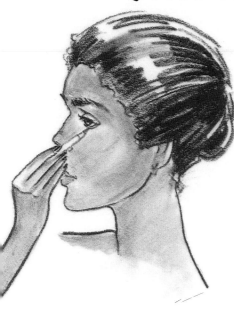

Curl your lashes with an eyelash curler. If you have the time, apply a brown, black, or colored mascara. Brush up your eyebrows and use eyebrow set or clear gloss over them.

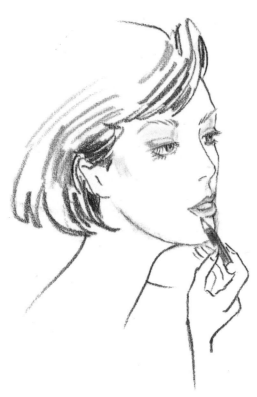

Next draw a thin line of pencil as close as possible to the lashes; smudge slightly with the thin tip of an applicator dipped in the same shade of cream or neon shadow. You may highlight the corners of the lid with pencil, as well, or draw an eye-opening line of kohl along the inner rim of the eye as a final, brightening touch.

Outline your natural lip line with a pencil and then put on gloss or lipstick. Use your lip brush to blend the lipstick into the line of pencil, so that the line disappears.

You're ready to go.

# CUTTING CORNERS

Any cosmetic in pencil form can be applied much more quickly than makeups that require brushes. Pencils have the additional advantage of being virtually mistake-proof.

Take a few seconds to curl your lashes with a curler; it opens your eyes without a fuss. Avoid mascara unless you have the time to apply it properly. If you tint your lashes periodically, you'll have a naturally dark frame and won't need the extra emphasis of mascara for your daytime makeups.

If you tint your brows as well, you also won't need to use an eyebrow pencil. Reshape eyebrows regularly and you can brush them up in seconds before using eyebrow set over them. Eyebrow set takes only a few seconds to apply, and its slightly shiny effect lasts all day.

# THE TAXI MAKEUP

Here's a makeup for days when you don't have time to put on makeup. All of us have done it—sat in the front of a car, the back of a taxi or a bus—and attempted to pull together a presentable look. After years of putting on makeup in transit, I've made a virtue out of necessity and perfected my taxi makeup. Its basis is your powder compact, a pocketbook essential.

When you have the time, by all means brush loose transparent powder over foundation. But when you don't—pressed powder goes on over moisturizer in seconds and functions as foundation and powder in one.

Press your powder puff *firmly* onto skin to create a foundation. Never rub. Dab concealer under each eye, then rub in cream blusher with your fingers (sponges are harder to control in heavy traffic). Blend blusher over eyelids and lips as well as cheeks. While you're safely stopped for a red light, outline the inside and outside of your eyes with two complementary shades of pencil and run a transparent gloss over your lips. When you arrive at your destination, you'll look—and feel—like a different person.

# TWO MINUTES TO GO

A sweater-and-jeans version of your five minutes' makeup can get you out of the house in half the time. Pare your makeup base down to a tinted moisturizer and concealer, than add a mousse blusher (which works well over a moisturizer because of its cream base), shadows, gloss, and pencils.

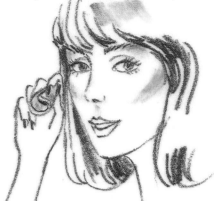

You can use any of the eye and lip makeups that work for your five-minute looks. Or try fast-acting cosmetics—for example, a line of kohl pencil drawn inside the eye is an instant eye makeup; add shadow for a complete eye look. Or double-duty makeups. One example is the mousse blusher you just put on your cheeks: a drop over the eye, another drop on the lips—blend and you have instant color.

And if you're literally racing out the door, use lipstick or gloss straight from the tube. You won't get the finished look you'll get with an outlining pencil and a brush, but you will have color.

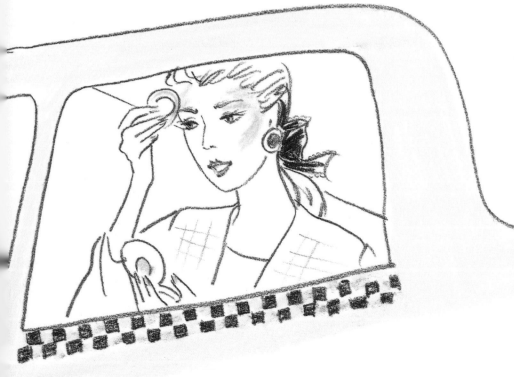

# MINIMAL MAKEUPS

No time? You can create a look—and an effective, interesting look—out of virtually nothing.

Use that invaluable fashion accessory, a pair of dark glasses, as the focus of the simplest summer makeup ever. The glasses liberate you from putting on eye makeup; all you have to do is put on tinted moisturizer, blusher, and lip makeup. The look works best if you team orange or red frames with a matching gloss or lipstick.

For another summery look, create a tanned appearance by brushing tan or bronze transparent powder over moisturized skin in a wide band over cheekbones and nose. Blend a line of jumbo eye pencil under lower lashes with a sponge-tip applicator to give the effect of a shadow. Add lip gloss and go.

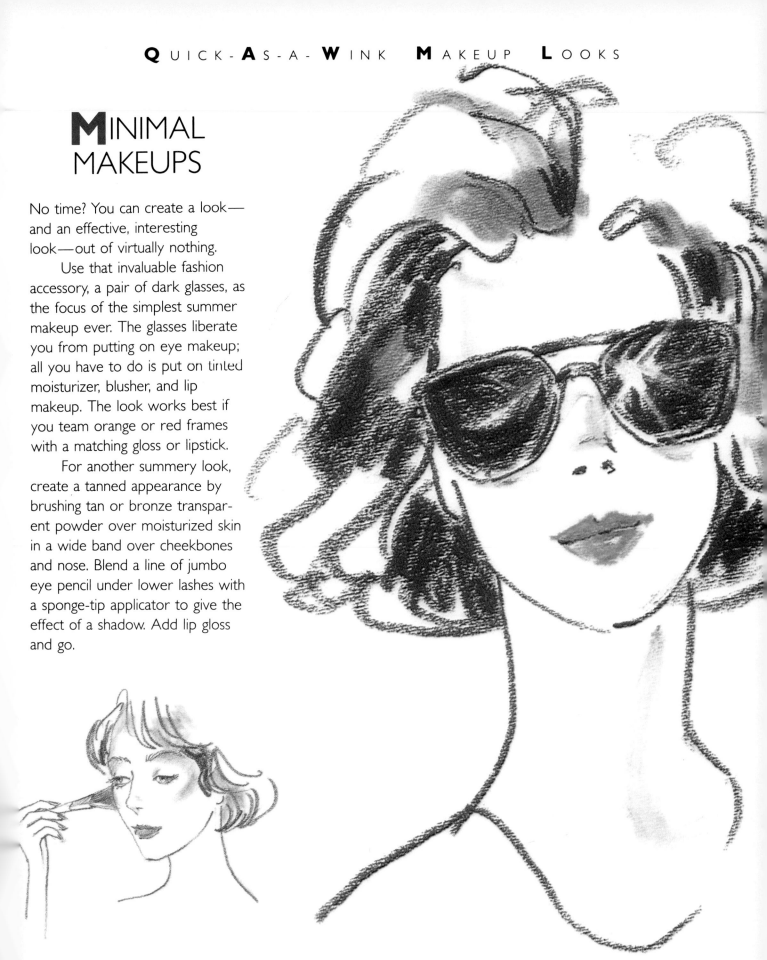

You can use powder blushers to create almost entire makeups. Choose one that will complement your natural skin tone and hair color: a reddish-brown, for instance, if you have red highlights in your hair; or a pink if you're a blonde. Blend blusher over a moisturizer base with a large brush and a light hand. Sweep color in a V-shape around each eye and then brush over the crease and on lips. For a little more color, blend whatever's left on your brush into your hairline and over your jawline. Outline the eye with pencil and blend in powder shadow with a sponge-tip applicator.

You can even create a makeup look without using makeup. When it's too hot to wear makeup, put on a sunscreen and pull out your lip balm. Coat the lips so they look shiny, then run lip balm over eyelids and under eyes so that the entire eye area is protected and has the hint of a sheen. Kohl eye pencil is an intriguing finishing touch.

# CHANGES— THIRTY SECONDS TO GO

Each of these changes takes seconds, yet each radically alters your appearance:

- Create an entire eye makeup in less than thirty seconds by using two shades of kohl pencil. Use the lighter shade to draw a line inside the rim of your eye, then put the darker pencil directly under your bottom lashes.
- For an instant eye makeup, use a sponge-tip applicator to blend a line of powder shadow on the lower part of your lid and in the area under your bottom lashes. For best results, sweep the flat end of your applicator under bottom lashes and use the rounded end on the lower part of your lid.
- Draw a thin line of eyeliner around the eye, keeping as close to the lashes as possible; your eye will look twice as large in seconds.
- Blend in rouge under eyebrows and over lips as well as on your cheeks.
- Another one-color idea: Blend an appropriate powder or cream shadow over your eyes and lips to focus attention equally on your two most compelling features.
- Or—outline lips and eyes with the same pencil.

# TOUCHUPS AFTER LUNCH— THIRTY SECONDS TO GO

- Carry a compact of foundation-colored pressed powder wherever you go. At the first hint of breakthrough shine (it appears first on nose and forehead), take your powder puff and pat on powder.
- To restore blusher color, use a pressed powder that blends in with your original blusher.
- Freshen lip color by adding lipstick or gloss.

## Double-Duty Concealer

You'd like to reshape your lips for an after-office party? You can do it using concealer and lip pencil. You want to revive your makeup? A touch of concealer under each eye will bring back your fast-fading look in seconds. Or use concealer as an eye highlighter by blending in below the brow line and on top of cheekbones. Concealer is a must for your thirty-second touchups.

# FROM OFFICE TO DINNER DATE IN FIVE MINUTES OR LESS

When you don't have time to go home and do a complete makeup before your evening out, you have to be a quick-change makeup artist. And the key to renewing your look is the long-lasting makeup base you put on in the morning: Leave it alone, it lasts all day.

Before adding new color, brush on transparent powder, making sure to powder eyelids and lips as well as cheeks, nose, and chin. Then add the finishing touches:

- Reshape your lips to look fuller.
- Put on new lip shades; combine two lipstick colors or a gloss and a lipstick for your after-hours look.
- Choose a color shadow to match your main accessory for the evening. Use as a highlighter or, if you wish, as your principal shadow. Since it reflects the color of your predominant accessory, it can pull your entire look together.

- Use mascara as the focus of your makeup. Choose a mascara color that gives a dark frame to the eyes, then heighten the effect (drawing attention away from your lips toward your eyes) by using a pale color on your lips. Or create a one-color eye makeup with mascara and a matching pencil: black on black for drama; blue on blue for excitement.

# CHAPTER SEVEN

# **G**UIDE TO A **P**ROFESSIONAL- **L**OOKING **M**AKEUP

Makeup is an art of almost infinite variations on a theme. The colors you choose may create looks as different from each other as day from night, and specific cosmetic choices (choosing a cream rather than a powder blusher, for example, or a gloss instead of a lipstick) can also provide intriguing alternatives, but the basics remain the same. This chapter will provide you with those basics—an illustrated step-by-step guide to a long-lasting, professional-looking makeup.

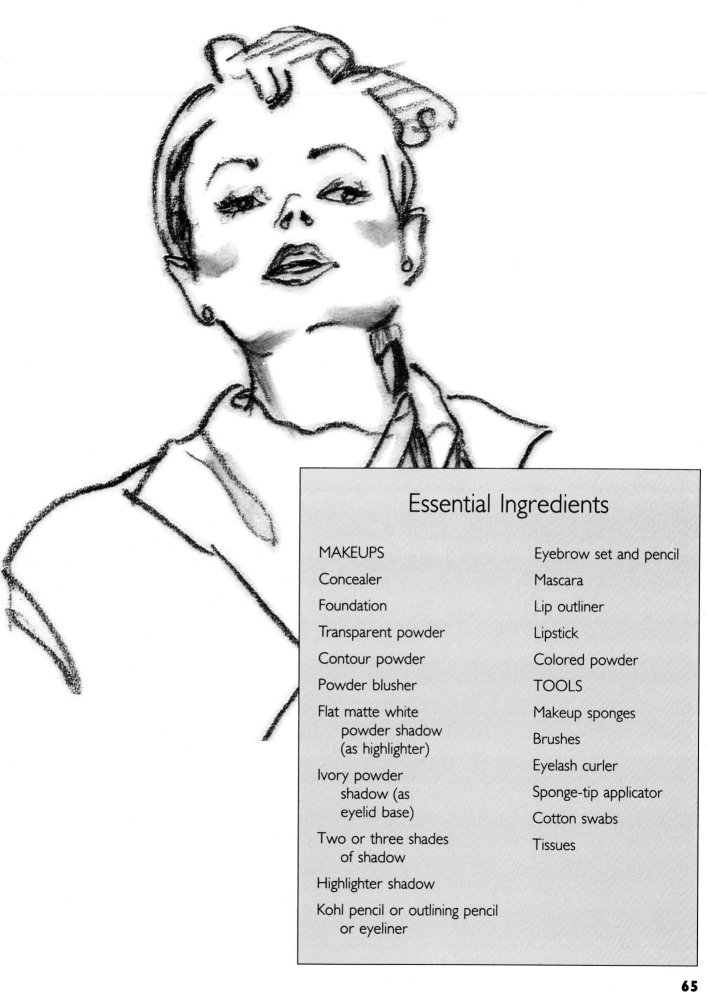

## Essential Ingredients

MAKEUPS

Concealer

Foundation

Transparent powder

Contour powder

Powder blusher

Flat matte white
powder shadow
(as highlighter)

Ivory powder
shadow (as
eyelid base)

Two or three shades
of shadow

Highlighter shadow

Kohl pencil or outlining pencil
or eyeliner

Eyebrow set and pencil

Mascara

Lip outliner

Lipstick

Colored powder

TOOLS

Makeup sponges

Brushes

Eyelash curler

Sponge-tip applicator

Cotton swabs

Tissues

# BEFORE YOU BEGIN

If you want to create a beautiful, long-lasting makeup, it's essential to start on clean, fresh skin. Residue—dirt from the environment as well as oils from your own system—collects on the skin and should be removed before you start applying makeup. After cleansing with a product specially formulated for your skin type, you should use a tonic (if you have oily skin) or a moisturizer. You may even need an astringent lotion *and* a moisturizer: tonic on an oily T-zone and moisturizer everywhere else.

Apply moisturizer in a three-dot pattern (three on each cheek, three on your forehead, two on your nose, and one on your chin) to ensure even coverage. Also apply on eyelids and over lips. Be careful not to use too much, and blend well so that your skin will be sealed and protected from the ravages of nature and pollution.

Now you are ready to begin putting on your makeup.

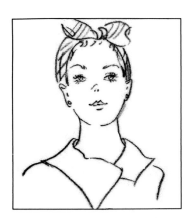

# SIXTEEN STEPS TO A COMPLETE MAKEUP LOOK

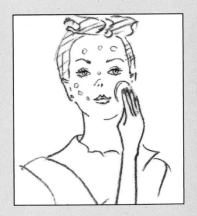

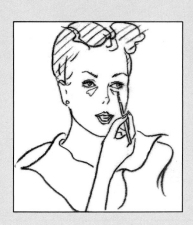

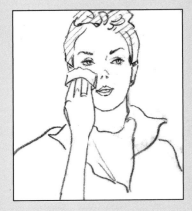

**1. Concealer** Using a cotton swab or a small brush, draw a line of concealer around the inner corner of your eye. Blend well; there should be no line of demarcation when concealer is properly blended into the skin. Then blend concealer down from the side of your mouth to cover smile lines, between the eyebrows to cover frown marks, around nostrils to hide broken capillaries, and over blemishes—wherever needed.

**2. Foundation** Put a few drops of foundation onto a dry makeup sponge and distribute on your face in a three-dot pattern. Blend quickly in long, even strokes down toward the jawline and up to the hairline, until forehead and cheeks are covered. Using a corner of your sponge, dab hard-to-reach areas around your nose, mouth, and chin. Blend your makeup base into your lips, then apply one more dot to each eyelid. Stroke the skin around the eye gently as you work the foundation inward. Check coverage, dabbing with your sponge until imperfections have disappeared.

Finally, blot with a tissue to remove excess foundation or any oily residue.

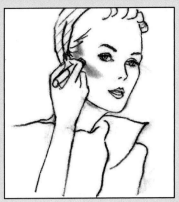

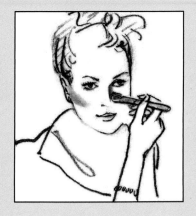

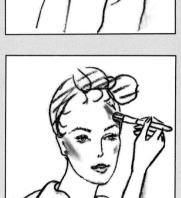

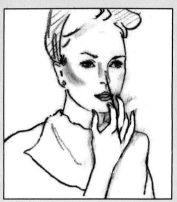

**3.** **Loose Transparent Powder** Sprinkle your basic shade of loose transparent powder into the palm of your hand. Lightly dip your powder brush into the powder and dab over cheeks, chin, nose, and forehead, then brush over eyelids and lips. Use more powder to cover oily skin; less if your skin is dry.

**4.** **Contour** Use your straight-edged contour or blusher brush to apply a dark-toned contour powder. (Remember, light emphasizes, dark recedes.) The same general technique applies wherever you use contour. Draw a line of contour powder over the area you wish to shade, then blend until the line becomes a shadow.

In applying contour to cheeks, jaw, forehead, temples, and so forth, think oval: Shorten a long face, narrow a round face to give your face a more perfect shape. When applying contour to your cheeks, blend contour in a downward direction from the line directly under your cheekbone, thus causing the hollow of the cheek to recede in relation to the height of the bone. Apply to the sides of your nose to narrow it; complete the illusion by drawing a thin line of concealer down the center of the nose. Contour under your chin to mask a double chin. Apply down the sides of your neck to elongate your neck. In short, use contour wherever you need it—and blend, always blend, until the line of powder becomes a shadow.

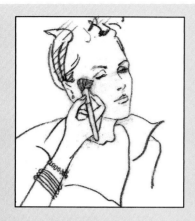

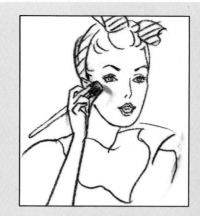

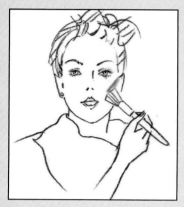

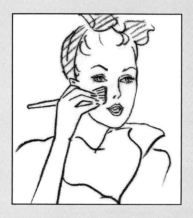

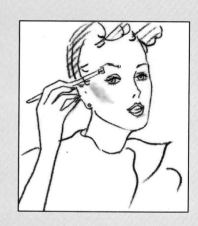

## 5.
**Blusher** Dip a blusher brush in a powder blusher and shake off the excess. Draw a line of color directly under your cheekbones and right on top of your contour shadow. Blend in an upward direction; the brighter blusher shade will stand out in contrast to the darker contour below, thus accentuating the height of the cheekbone. Blend until the line becomes a shadow and there is no clear line delineating contour from blusher.

## 6.
**Cheek Highlighter** Use a flat matte white powder shadow as a cheek highlighter. Dip your powder brush into the shadow and draw a line of highlighter just above the line of your blusher. The line will visually separate your cheekbone from your eye. Next create a rough triangle of highlighter all around your cheekbone and under the line of contour to further pronounce the height of your cheekbone. Blend until the lines become shadows.

## 7.
**Eyelid Base** Use your flat brush to smooth an ivory-colored powder shadow all the way from your brows to your top lashes. This shadow will even the color of your skin and absorb oiliness and perspiration that could affect your color shadows. Blend in well before applying other shadows.

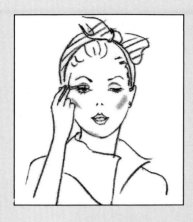

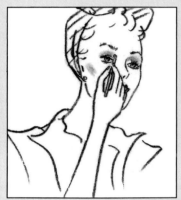

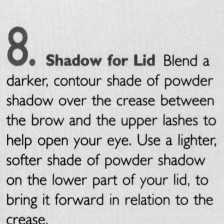

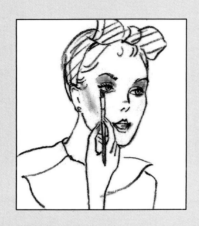

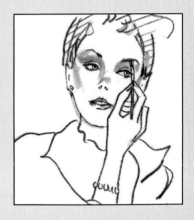

**8.** **Shadow for Lid** Blend a darker, contour shade of powder shadow over the crease between the brow and the upper lashes to help open your eye. Use a lighter, softer shade of powder shadow on the lower part of your lid, to bring it forward in relation to the crease.

**9.** **Shadow Under Bottom Lashes** Use a darker shadow (either the same shade as on the crease or another dark shade) under the bottom lashes. It will cause this potentially puffy area to recede in relation to the areas around it.

**10.** **Highlighter Shadow Under Brows** Use a lightcolored flat matte powder shadow or an iridescent shadow to highlight the area between the brow bone and the crease. Needless to say, all your shadows should be blended so that they almost melt into one another; *you should never be able to tell where one shadow ends and the next begins.*

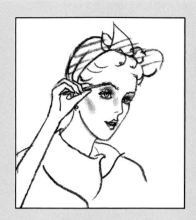

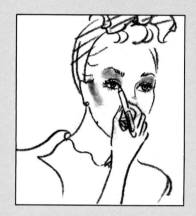

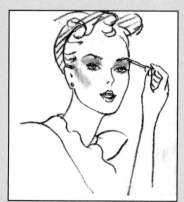

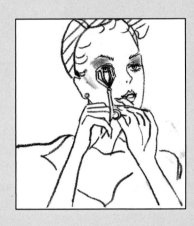

**11.** **Pencil or Eyeliner** Pick up a thick, soft kohl pencil, look down, and gently pull down your bottom lashes before placing your pencil inside the rim of your eye. Draw a pencil line inside and all around the eye. The almost invisible line will markedly increase the apparent size of your eye.

Alternatively, use a big outlining pencil to draw a line around the eye. Hold at an angle and keep as close as possible to the lashes. Blend your pencil line into your powder shadows with a sponge-tip applicator.

Another, more dramatic alternative is eyeliner. Wet your eyeliner brush, dip it in cake liner, and apply the liner as close as possible to the lashes.

**12.** **Eyebrows** For a natural brow look, first brush your brows up, then color with pencil. Use a taupe pencil for fair brows and a charcoal for dark brows (or an auburn if you have reddish highlights in your hair). Holding your pencil at an angle, apply between the hairs with short, light pencil strokes. Then take your applicator brush and brush on eyebrow set, to keep your eyebrow look in place for hours.

**13.** **Eyelash Curler** Keeping your eye open, gently place your eyelash curler midway over your top lashes. Press for about thirty seconds and release.

**70**

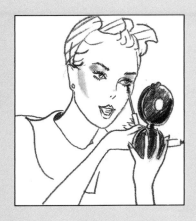

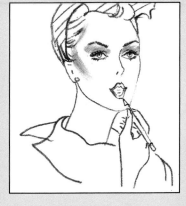

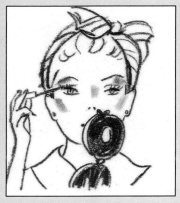

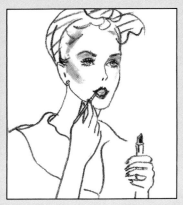

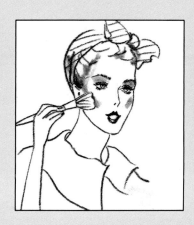

**14.** **Mascara** Start with the bottom lashes, and roll your applicator up and down the curl of the lashes with a very light touch. Allow a few seconds to dry before you start on your top lashes. Start with the top of your upper lashes, rolling your wand right up the curl of your lashes before gently stroking the ends. Repeat on the inside to exaggerate the curl.

**15.** **Lip Outline** Outline your lips with a soft pencil or a lip brush. Place a dot of liner at each peak of your Cupid's bow and two more spots of color directly underneath at the bottom of your lower lip line. Trace your lip line between the dots with liner. Then complete lining by working color in from the corners of your mouth. (Attempting to line your lips with one continuous line is bound to make you waver!)

Use a lip brush to stroke color onto your lips. For a fuller appearance, leave the center of your lips open and fill in with a matching gloss. Blend with your brush.

**16.** **Colored Powder** As a finishing touch, add a colorful glow to your makeup by fluffing on a colored or tinted transparent powder. Use a firmer hand over a potentially oily T-zone area to prevent breakthrough shine later. Brush over your forehead, around the jawline, and over your eyelids and lips, using a lighter hand wherever your skin is dry.

# CHAPTER EIGHT

# SPECIAL OCCASIONS, SPECIAL EFFECTS

There are occasions in every woman's life when she has the time, the energy, the wherewithal, the desire—and even the need—to let her imagination take wing. These special occasions call for special effects: sophisticated, playful, sometimes outrageous makeup. Glitter gel, false eyelashes, a virtual rainbow of iridescent dusts and more; makeups in all the colors of your fantasies. I love them!

If you're in a hurry, save your special effects makeup for another time. Nightplay is fun, and getting there, indulging yourself in creating a glittering new sophisticated look, should be a savored pleasure. So relax, pamper yourself; it may take an hour, even two, to complete your special effects makeup. But every minute can be a

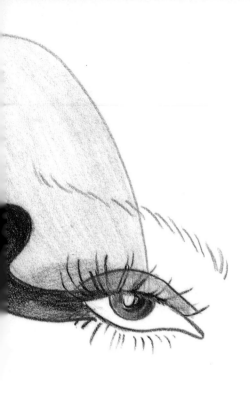
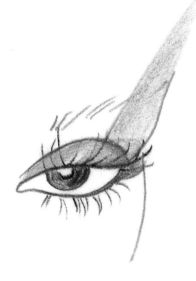
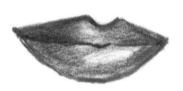

## Special Effects

Add these to your basic steps.

MAKEUPS
Toner

Two shades of blusher

Kohl pencil

Eye pencils

Top and bottom strip
eyelashes or individual
top and bottom lashes

Eyeliner

Glitters

Glitter gel

Highlighter dust

Eyebrow set

Liquid shimmer

Colored rhinestones

TOOLS

Small cardboard wedge

Eyelash glue

Wedge-shaped brush for
eyeliner

delight if your mood fits the occasion and the occasion is something special.

In the following pages, I'll explain one particular special effects makeup look; in "The Many Looks of You," Part 2 of this book, you'll see examples of nine more. But the possibilities are endless: Remember, your clean face is like a fresh canvas; let your imagination take you!

# A LUMINOUS AND LIGHT SPECIAL EFFECTS LOOK

"Special" can mean many things, but in this particular case it means ethereal. Of course, there are many bolder, stronger night looks, but this makeup is luminous, based on sheer, shimmering cosmetics for lips and eyes.

## The Makeup Base

To show sheer lip and eye makeups to their best advantage, create a very light background by mixing foundation a shade lighter than your skin with a few drops of white toner. It's an effect I wouldn't recommend for day, but it looks like a dream in the evening. (If you're black, simply use foundation a shade or two lighter than your skin; you don't need toner.)

First use concealer, then the foundation/toner mixture and finally a loose powder that matches the foundation.

### Eyedrops

Any occasion, but particularly a special one, calls for clear eyes. If your eyes are tired and dry, or if the little blood vessels in them are peeking through, refresh and clarify them with eyedrops before putting on your makeup. Your eyes will sparkle—and so will you.

## Blusher and Contour

Use two tones of a similar shade of blusher, one lighter (such as a pink or a peach) and one darker (perhaps a rose or a coral). Apply the darker rouge under the cheekbone as a contour, then blend the lighter shade directly above. The result is a light, subtly shaded, monochromatic blusher look.

## Eye Shadow

To get a strikingly light eye look, create a halo of shadow that extends way beyond the usual eye shadow boundaries, all around the eyes and up into the brows as well. The effect—positively luminous.

First create the upward motion of the eye color. Feather the eyebrows by brushing the hairs up and out with a small stiff brush to slightly separate the hairs. Then brush a line of shadow over the crease of the eye and blend it up, right into the brows.

Next extend the shadow out.
Here you can use a simple airbrush card trick, which has the effect of magic but is hardly sleight-
of-hand. Cut a small wedge out of
cardboard, then place it on its side
at a 45-degree angle to the ridge
of your cheekbone. Now brush a
line of shadow in an outward direction until you reach the end of
the card.

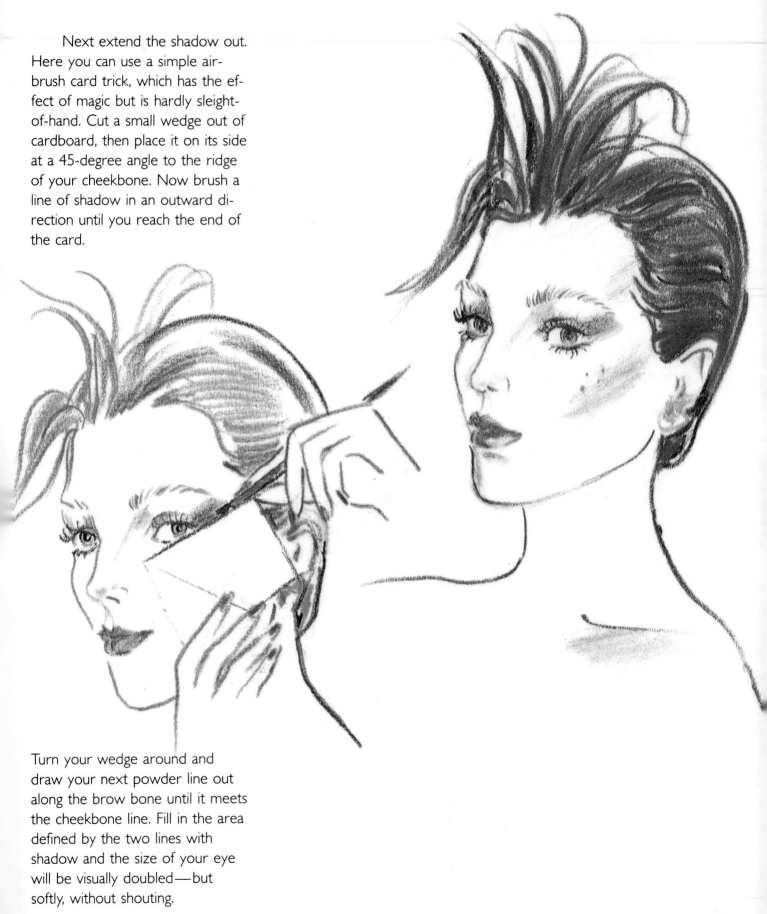

Turn your wedge around and
draw your next powder line out
along the brow bone until it meets
the cheekbone line. Fill in the area
defined by the two lines with
shadow and the size of your eye
will be visually doubled—but
softly, without shouting.

## Pencils and Eyeliner

Use a shade of pencil that is darker than your shadow to smudge a faint accent into the corners of the eyes.

Run a line of kohl pencil around the rim of the eye to further expand your eye and to brighten the effect.

To add to the dramatic effect of your eye, draw a line of black eye pencil as close to the lashes as possible.

To create even stronger eye definition, draw a thin line of cake eyeliner directly over your pencil line.

## Eyelashes

Adding extra lashes can add to the fun of your special effects eye makeup.

Always curl your lashes and put on mascara before adding strip lashes. Curling your own lashes can help you match the curl of the strip lashes, and mascara is almost impossible to put on over false lashes. To maintain the silvery look of this makeup use a black mascara rather than brown or a color.

Using tweezers, delicately pick up your **strip lashes** on the outer corner of the strip. Before you begin applying lashes, try them against your natural lashes for size and length. If you haven't bought precut lashes, cut the ends to fit.

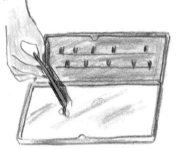

To apply strip lashes, squeeze eyelash glue along the top of the strip. Grasp lashes in the center and, rounding them a little at the ends, look down and attach lashes at the center, easing the ends toward the corners of your eye. Your mascara will help bond the false lashes to your natural lashes for a completely snug fit.

To cover the "line" created by the false lashes, dip your brush in glitter gel and draw a thin line over your eyelid. Glitter gel is more intensely "glittery" than standard iridescent shadows; subdued artificial lighting reflects its sparkle beautifully.

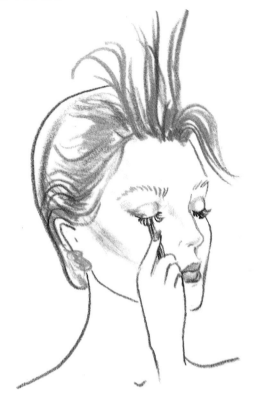

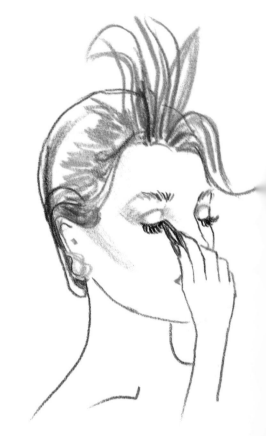

**Individual or cluster lashes** are an alternative to strip lashes; they give you the option of putting on as many lashes as you want. To apply them you need surgical glue and tweezers.

For an especially dramatic look, use mascara before putting on cluster lashes.

To apply: Squeeze a small pool of glue onto the plastic case that holds your lashes; point tweezers across tips of lashes toward the bulb of the cluster and pick up lashes as close to the bulb as possible; dip the bulb into the glue; hold the cluster against your lashes (since placement is the key to a natural-looking result, get as close to the rim of the lid as you can without touching it); apply the cluster. You will be applying your cluster lashes twice: the first time to reshape your eye and the second time to add thickness. In the first application, put lashes on from the outside of one eye all the way across to the outside of the other. The second time, alternate eyes to ensure evenness of application, adding lashes until you've arrived at the desired effect.

Lashes designed for the lower lid are more truly "individual" than the small clusters made for the top lid. Apply them one at a time until you've achieved the look you want.

## Lips

After shaping your lips with outlining pencil, try one of these combinations of lipstick and gloss to complete your ethereal look. Apply the same shade of lipstick to both top and bottom lips, either filling in the center of the lower lip or leaving it bare (to be covered later by gloss), or use different lip colors on top and bottom. You might apply gloss only in the center of your lips, either over lipstick or bare foundation, or try using a gloss that's a different color from your lipstick. The gloss will give a glow and also pleasantly plump the appearance of your mouth.

To further accent your luminescent total look, add highlighter dust over your gloss: iridescents to complement sheer shadows, for example, or ultraviolet if your shadows are blue.

## Finishing Touches

Rub glitter gel on your fingers; run fingers through your hair so your hair catches the glitter.

Put liquid shimmer on top of your cheekbone as a highlighter. It will give your skin a high gloss.

Sprinkle sparkling highlighter dust on the ridge of your cheekbones; your face will seem to catch on fire as it reflects the light.

Use eyelash glue and tweezers to put colored rhinestones on your cheek, your chest, anywhere your heart desires.

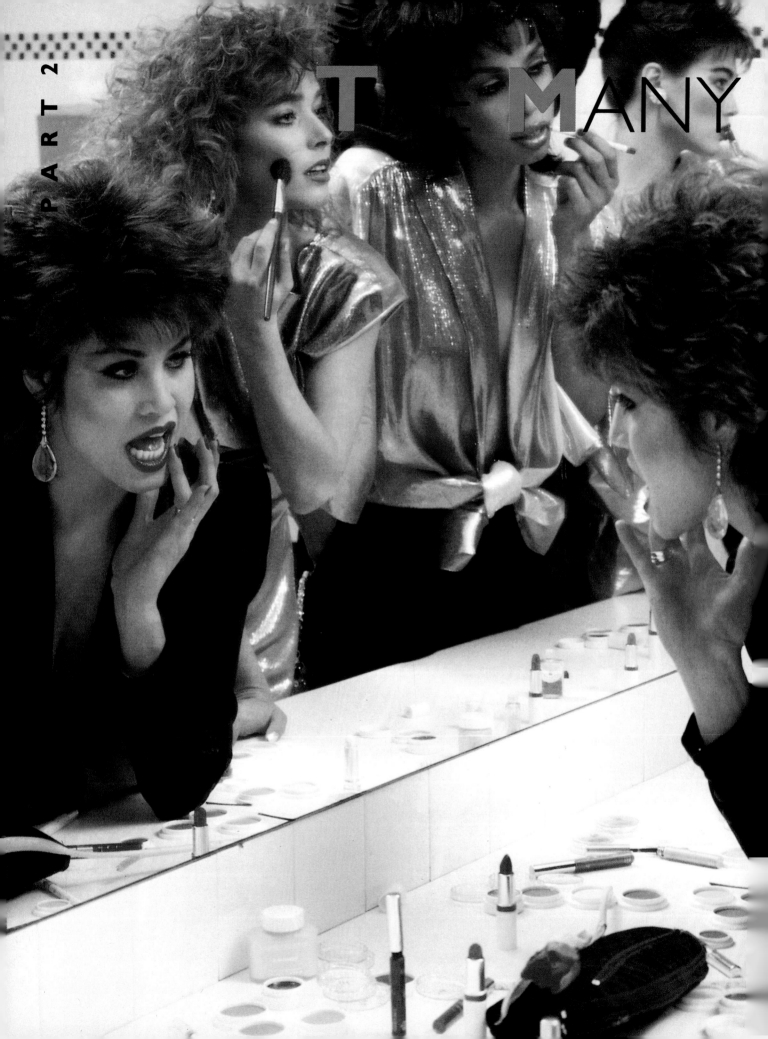

# PART 2

TOO MANY

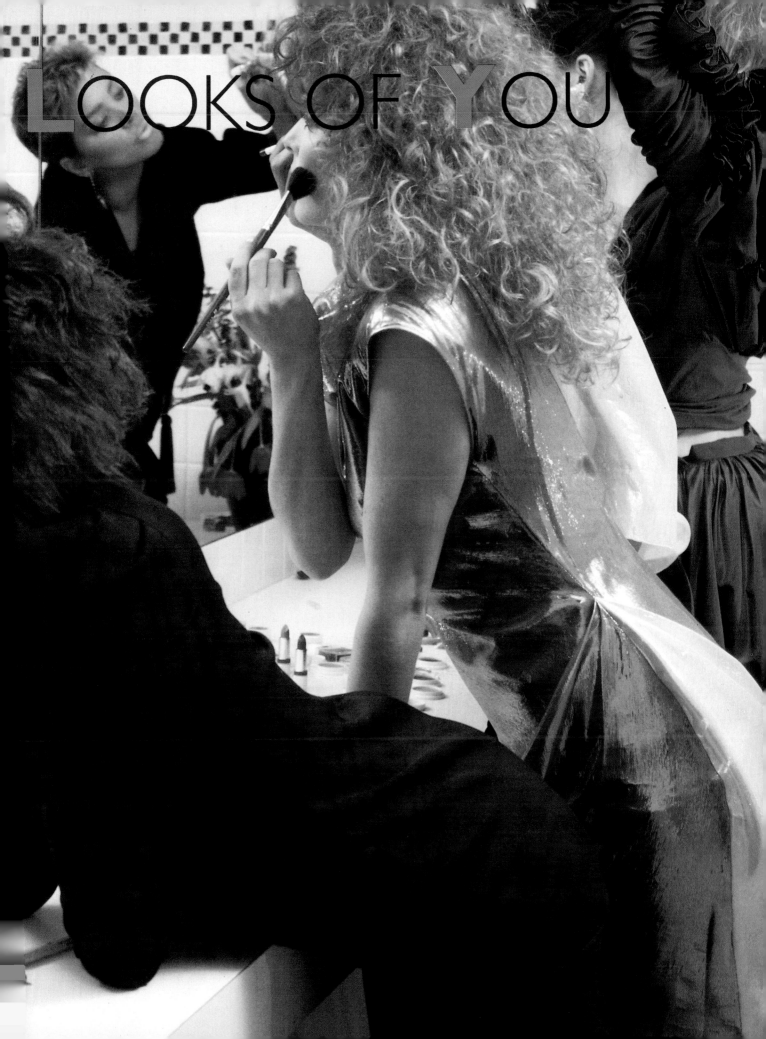

# LOOKS OF YOU

In "The Makeup Lesson" I described how you can transform your look to fit your mood, how you can rise to any occasion smashingly, how you can break the color barrier. But sometimes, I know, words and sketches are not enough; seeing is believing. And that's why I've created "The Many Looks of You": I want you to see exactly how any woman can change her look, superchange her natural beauty, and be whoever she wants to be.

I've chosen nine models, each unique—with a personality, complexion, hair and eye color, and features unlike any of the others. Along the way to discovering their many looks, six of them break the color barrier either subtly or spectacularly. Among the others, one was chosen to showcase the range and drama of monochromatic moods, another to demonstrate the principles of balance in makeup, and one to display the fresh and colorful makeup variation appropriate to a more mature beauty. The common thread between them (*and you*) is that they are all multifaceted personalities whose different moods and activities can be heightened and enlivened by the creative use of makeup and its coordination with clothing and accessories. Those myriad possibilities inherent in every woman—the possibilities that keep life exciting—have been made real by these photographs.

You may see parts of yourself in one or another of these women, or you may see a makeup look that you would like to try for yourself. To enable you to do so, I've included detailed information about each of the makeups I've chosen, so that you can re-create a look or a combination of colors that you particularly like.

These photos represent not only new ways of seeing other women, but new ways of seeing yourself—as a person whose beauty possibilities are as limitless and surprising as each new day.

# LA DOLCE VITA

Caroline has classic features: beautiful, deepset eyes, prominent cheekbones...and an aura of natural sophistication.

We chose her to illustrate how a woman can project unlimited looks and levels of sophistication by working primarily with her basic colors and accents of

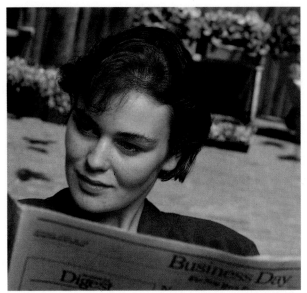

a much broader spectrum. Caroline has brown hair, fair skin, and hazel-green eyes; she always looks good in warm browns, yellows, oranges, and greens. We stretched her color options by adding fuchsias, lavenders, pinks, and blues to her palette, providing variations that allowed her to show, in turn, her natural intelligence, sophisticated finesse, and smoldering sensuality—all moods of the same complex woman.

Caroline's sensitive skin has a tendency toward redness and oily patches around the T-zone. With her complexion she needs regular facials as well as a good makeup base to even out her skin tones. And with her natural coloring, just a little touch of henna brings out auburn highlights in her hair, immeasurably enhancing her total look.

**BEFORE:** Even without makeup Caroline's bone structure is striking. Her chiseled cheekbones draw your eyes to hers, which are soft and expressive. But her face is capable of communicating so much more...

## WHAT TO USE

FOUNDATION: Medium Beige
POWDER: Beige
CHEEKBONE: Magenta
EYES: Eye Contour: Lavender; Eyelid: Inner Corner—Pale Pink Iridescent Shadow, Outer Corner—Lavender
MASCARA: Royal Blue
LIP OUTLINE: Soft Pink Pencil
LIPSTICK: Mauve

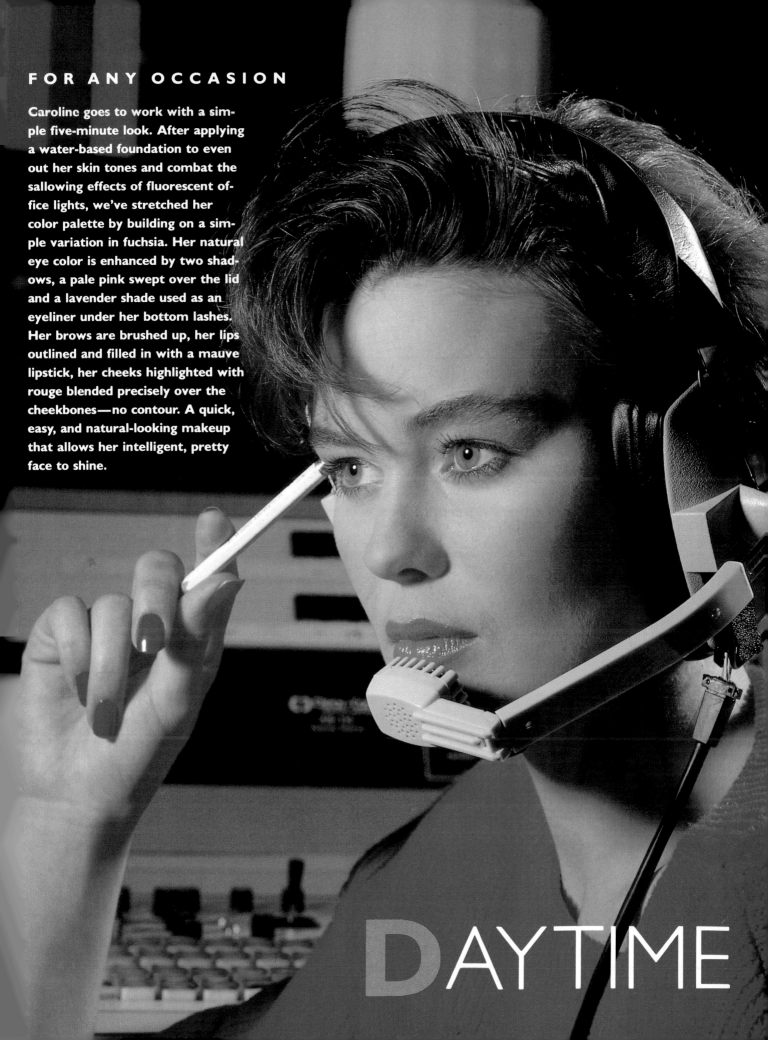

## FOR ANY OCCASION

Caroline goes to work with a simple five-minute look. After applying a water-based foundation to even out her skin tones and combat the sallowing effects of fluorescent office lights, we've stretched her color palette by building on a simple variation in fuchsia. Her natural eye color is enhanced by two shadows, a pale pink swept over the lid and a lavender shade used as an eyeliner under her bottom lashes. Her brows are brushed up, her lips outlined and filled in with a mauve lipstick, her cheeks highlighted with rouge blended precisely over the cheekbones—no contour. A quick, easy, and natural-looking makeup that allows her intelligent, pretty face to shine.

# DAYTIME

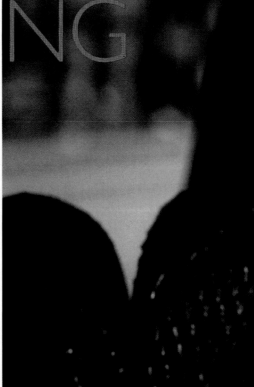

With a date right after work, Caroline's sophisticated evening look is built right on top of her five-minute daytime makeup. Her hair is pulled back, bringing her face forward and drawing attention to her eyes. Contour is used in conjunction with fuchsia rouge—on the sides of her forehead to narrow it, on the sides of her nose, along her cheekbones, and under her jawline. The contour helps create an elegant, chiseled look, increasing the impact of her dramatic eyes. We made her eyes appear more intensely green by blending fuchsia and blue tones over her lids. And where you might expect a dash of gold jewelry, the conventional complement to her eye color, we've added a spark of silver. So Caroline breaks her color barrier with accessories—and effectively creates a much more striking total look.

# EVENING

## WHAT TO USE

FOUNDATION: Medium Beige
POWDER: Beige/Violet (to finish)
CONTOUR: Under Cheekbone: White;
Jawline: Light Brown
CHEEKBONE: Fuchsia
CHEEKBONE HIGHLIGHTS: Pale Pink
Iridescent Dust
EYES: Eye Contour: Fuchsia; Eyelid: Inner
Corner—Pale Pink Iridescent Dust,
Outer Corner—Fuchsia
MASCARA: Black
BROW BONE: Fuchsia
LIP OUTLINE: Soft Pink Pencil
LIP GLOSS: Fuchsia (blended together
with pencil)

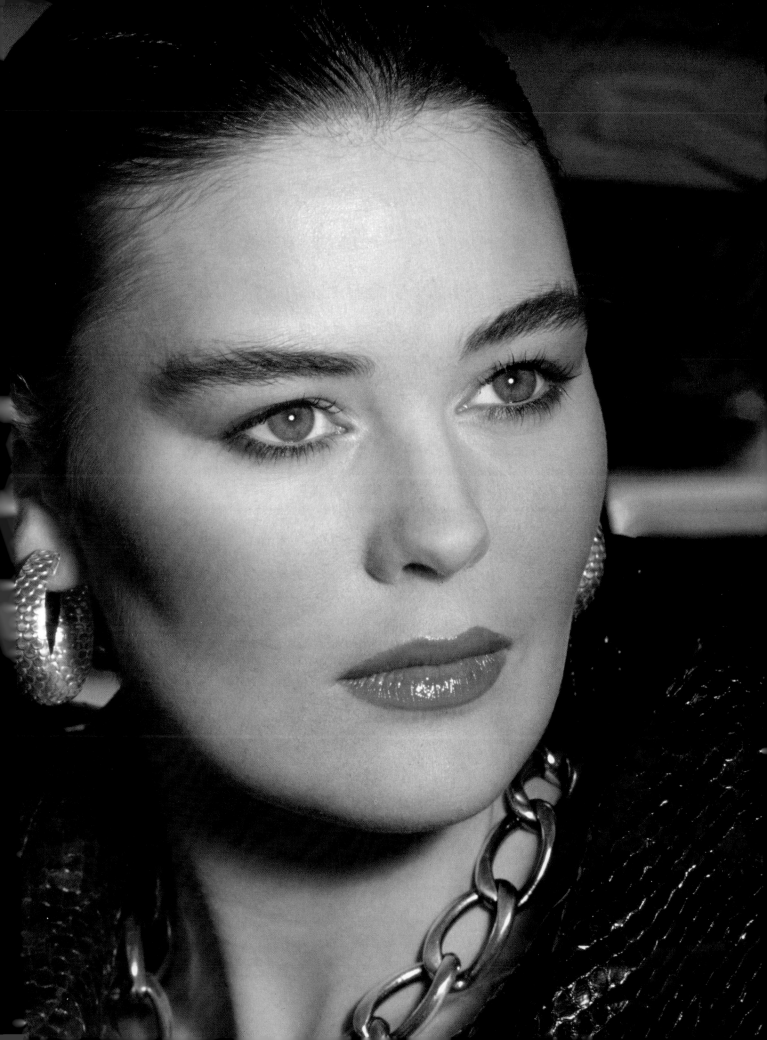

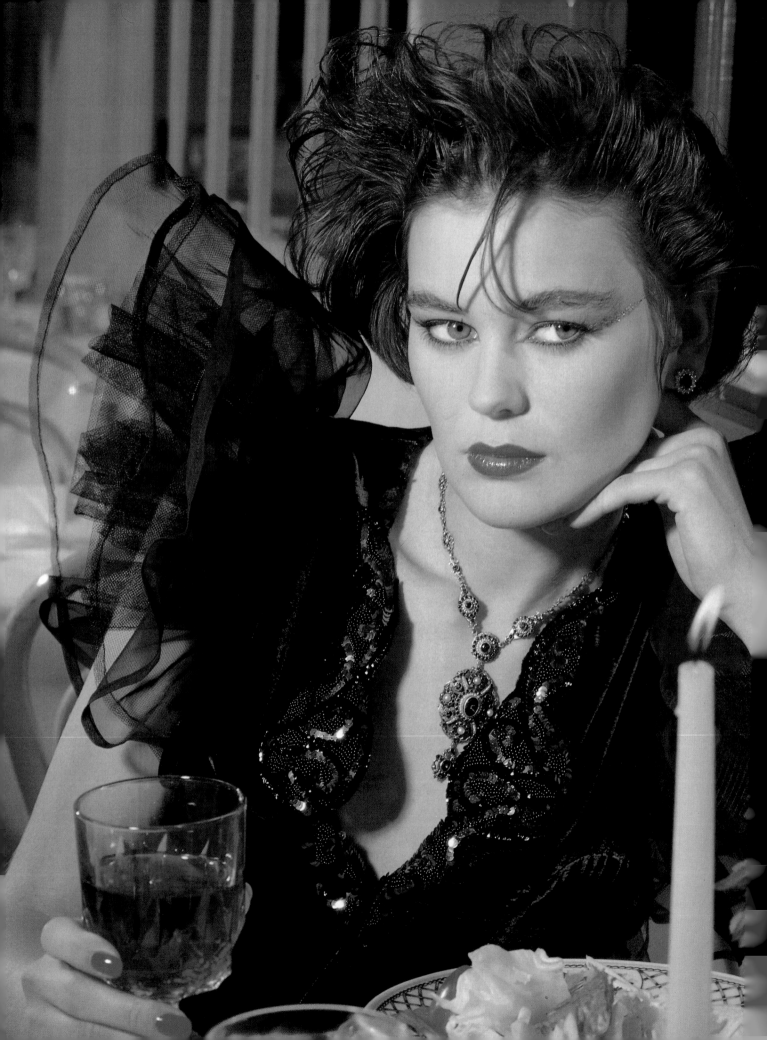

# NIGHTPLAY

Caroline's sultry, smoldering look is perfect for a candlelit dinner for two. We've sculpted her hair with a gel, and once again used blues to brighten the green of her eyes (highlighting them even more with special nightplay effects). After blending a bright blue shadow into the crease and under her bottom lashes, we created a powerful, almost masklike airbrush effect with a soft, narrow, pastel blue shadow line drawn diagonally up and out all the way to her hairline, using our card/airbrush technique. We then applied glitter right on the top of the line, using an eyeliner brush. Because Caroline's eyes are both deeply and widely set, we were able to use an indigo eyeliner all around her eye, even extending it inward to emphasize the inner corner. And we added fullness to her lashes with very short individual lashes.

The silvers, the blues, the cold tints with which we accented Caroline's look—all added to her overall effect of mystery and allure— irresistibly romantic.

## WHAT TO USE

FOUNDATION: Medium Beige
POWDER: Beige/Peach (to finish over contour areas)
CONTOUR: Under Cheekbone: Light Brown; Jawline: Magenta; Nose: Light Brown; Forehead: Magenta
CHEEKBONE: Magenta
CHEEKBONE HIGHLIGHTS: White Shadow
EYES: Eye Contour: Bright Blue; Eyeliner: Indigo Shadow (used wet), Blue Glitter Gel; Eyelid: Inner Corner—Ultra Violet Dust, Outer Corner—Bright Blue Shadow
MASCARA: Black
LIP OUTLINE: Beet Pencil
LIPSTICK: Hot Red
NAILS: Hot Red

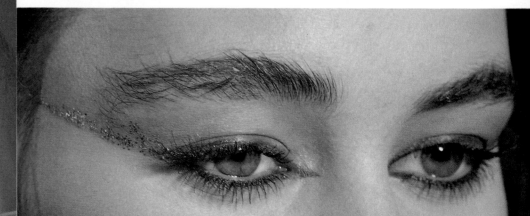

# THE PAMPERED BEAUTY

Lisa has striking individual features: full lips, a classic nose, big eyes, prominent cheekbones, and thick, expressive eyebrows. By accenting her features in different ways she can change her look nearly as easily as she changes clothes. And exploring her makeup options is exactly what we've done with her.

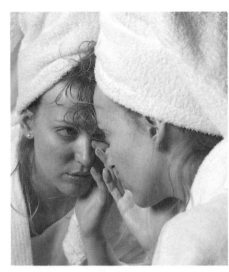

In these pages, Lisa's makeup ranges from a soft, innocent no-makeup look in natural earth tones to a fresh daytime scheme with dramatic accents to a makeup with exceptional impact and power. They're three very different effects with one critical aspect in common: balance—balance between eyes and lips; balance between makeup, clothes, hair, and accessories; and a balance of color and intensity.

Lisa's a strawberry blonde with the very fair and sensitive skin shared by many redheads. She can get broken capillaries in a hot shower, and needs to pamper and protect her skin. That's why I would always recommend that she use a foundation—both to protect her skin and to even out her skin tones. That way her stunning features can really shine through.

**BEFORE:**
**Lisa's skin shows the effects of a hot shower. Once the redness is toned down, her beauty can be brought out by emphasizing her lips, her cheekbones, her large, luminous eyes...**

## WHAT TO USE

FOUNDATION: Sheer Beige
POWDER: Peach and Beige mixed together
CONTOUR: Forehead: Apricot
CHEEKBONE: Apricot
NOSE HIGHLIGHTS: Apricot
EYELID BASE: Apricot
EYELINER: Coconut Pencil
MASCARA: Brown
EYEBROWS: Auburn Pencil/Brow Set
LIP OUTLINE: Ginger Pencil
LIP GLOSS: Apricot

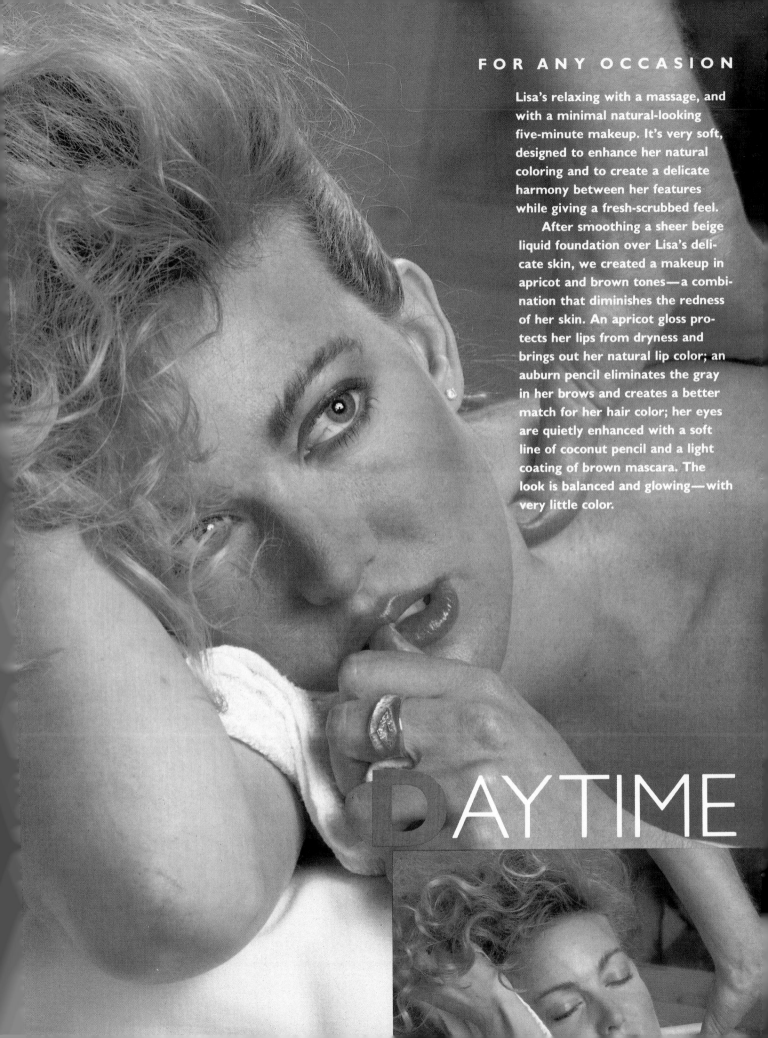

## FOR ANY OCCASION

Lisa's relaxing with a massage, and with a minimal natural-looking five-minute makeup. It's very soft, designed to enhance her natural coloring and to create a delicate harmony between her features while giving a fresh-scrubbed feel.

After smoothing a sheer beige liquid foundation over Lisa's delicate skin, we created a makeup in apricot and brown tones—a combination that diminishes the redness of her skin. An apricot gloss protects her lips from dryness and brings out her natural lip color; an auburn pencil eliminates the gray in her brows and creates a better match for her hair color; her eyes are quietly enhanced with a soft line of coconut pencil and a light coating of brown mascara. The look is balanced and glowing—with very little color.

# DAYTIME

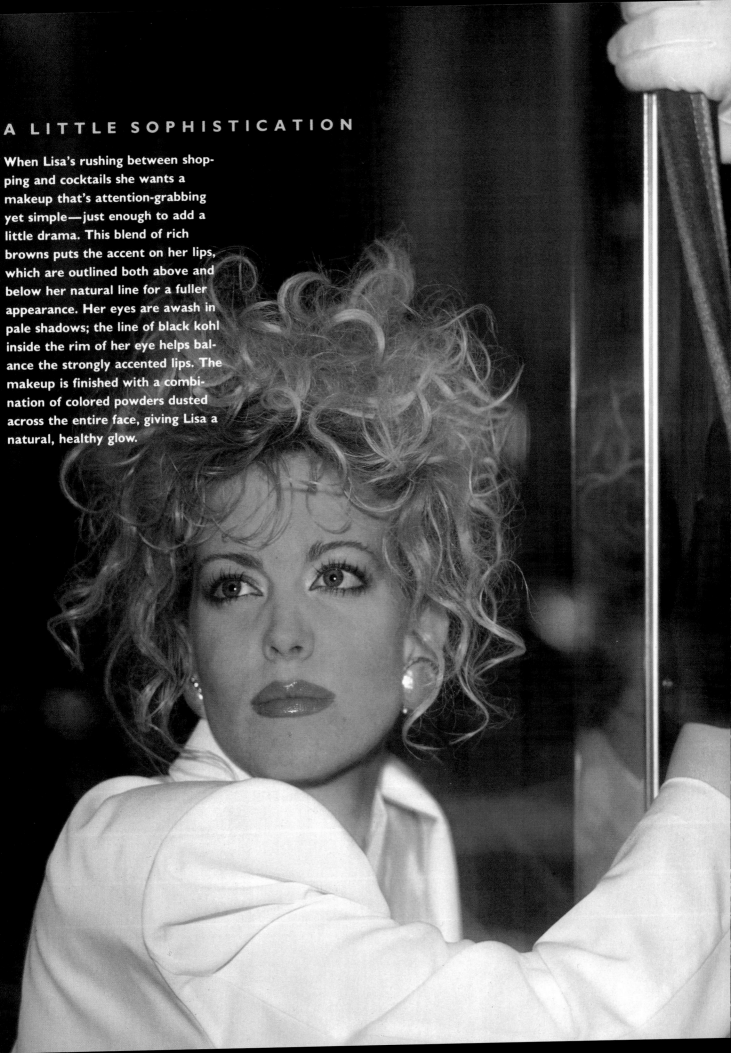

# A LITTLE SOPHISTICATION

When Lisa's rushing between shopping and cocktails she wants a makeup that's attention-grabbing yet simple—just enough to add a little drama. This blend of rich browns puts the accent on her lips, which are outlined both above and below her natural line for a fuller appearance. Her eyes are awash in pale shadows; the line of black kohl inside the rim of her eye helps balance the strongly accented lips. The makeup is finished with a combination of colored powders dusted across the entire face, giving Lisa a natural, healthy glow.

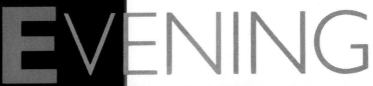

# EVENING

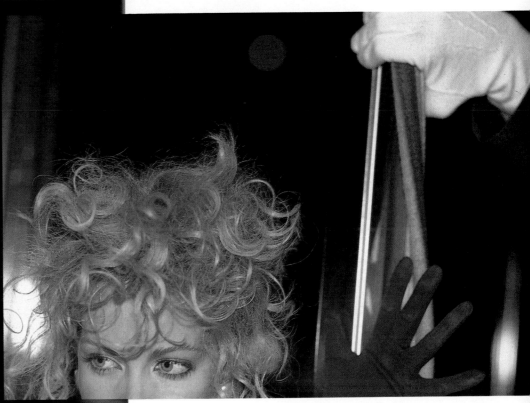

**WHAT TO USE**

FOUNDATION: Sheer Beige
POWDER: Peach and Bronze mixed together
CONTOUR: Under Cheekbone: White; Jawline: Indian Curry; Nose: Indian Curry
CHEEKBONE: Indian Curry
EYES: Eyeliner: Brown Cake Liner; Kohl Ebony Pencil (inside eye); Eyelid: Inner Corner—Mustard, Outer Corner—Camel
MASCARA: Black
EYEBROWS: Camel Shadow; Brow Set (optional)
LIP OUTLINE: Auburn Pencil
LIPSTICK: Soft Brown
LIP GLOSS: Clear (in center)

Lisa's fur, her jewelry, her wild flowing hair—they're all so intense that they would overwhelm a lightly made-up pretty face. A maximum makeup draws admiring eyes back to the center of attention—Lisa's expressive face.

Here we've given Lisa heavier coverage to even out her skin tone, neutralize the red undertone, and leave her with a natural-looking, porcelain finish. We then added rouge and contour to highlight and accent, but not to change the natural shape of Lisa's jawline, cheekbone, forehead, and nose.

And we made Lisa's eyes the most powerful element, the magnet of the makeup, by first lining with smoky black powder shadow, then shaping with a line of black liquid eyeliner. Blue glitter gel drawn over shadow and liner complete the frame. It's an extra-

# NIGHTPLAY

ordinarily bold combination (and one that only works because it's part of such a powerful total look).

But that's not all we did: We added black mascara; we contoured with black shadow in the crease; we defined Lisa's brows with a combination of brown charcoal shadow and, directly beneath, a soft line of pale pink rouge to emphasize their shape. Then we outlined Lisa's lips with a hot-pink pencil and filled them in with gypsy-red color. And as a finishing touch, we sprinkled gold highlighter dust over her eyes, her cheeks, her lips, and even her hair. A fourteen-karat look!

## WHAT TO USE

FOUNDATION: Sunny Beige Liquid Base
POWDER: Beige
CONTOUR: Under Cheekbone: Light Brown; Jawline: Light Brown; Nose: Light Brown
CHEEKBONE: Pale Pink
CHEEKBONE HIGHLIGHTS: Gold Dust
EYES: Eye Contour: Black; Eyeliner: Black Liquid, Blue Glitter Gel; Eyelid: Inner Corner—Gold Dust, Outer Corner—Black Shadow; Eye Highlights: Pale Pink
MASCARA: Black
EYEBROWS: Charcoal Brown
LIP OUTLINE: Hot Pink
LIPSTICK: Hot Red
LIP HIGHLIGHT: Gold Dust
HAIR HIGHLIGHT: Gold Dust

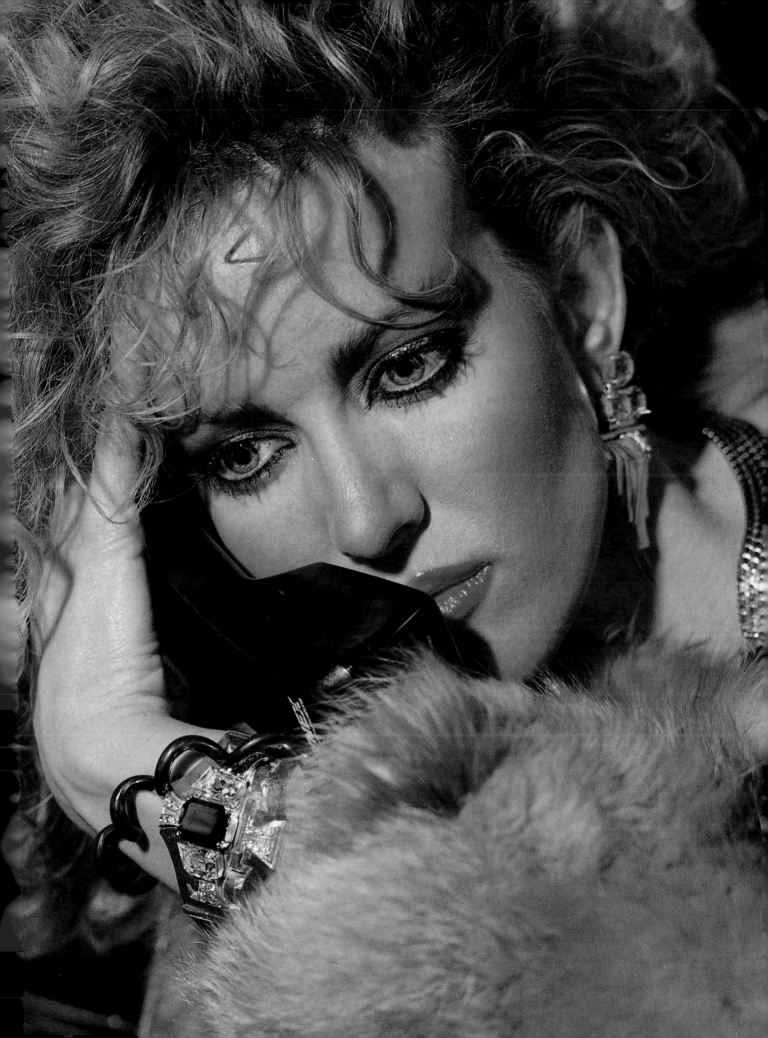

# JADE:

# ORIENTAL SUNRISE

Jade's deep eyes are the windows to her strong character. Her exotic look and her beautiful glowing skin are the keys to unlocking her unique beauty.

I chose her as a model to demonstrate how a person with yellow-toned skin can break the color barrier. Many women of Mediterranean or Oriental coloration feel limited in their color choices; even professional makeup artists have long felt constrained in dealing with color for the sallow complexion. But study the photos and you will see that the makeups I chose for Jade explode many myths about color. And the best news is that by preparing the skin properly, *anyone* can break the color barrier and wear cold or warm shades (or even a combination of the two); anyone can wear color makeups based on totally different, even contrasting families of colors; and every woman has unlimited color possibilities.

Jade, like many Orientals, has a relatively flat nose at the bridge, narrow eyes, and yellow-toned skin. Her most effective makeups widen her eyes and give more definition to the shape of her nose. They also bring out the moods of a woman whose inner strength and mystery simmer just beneath the surface.

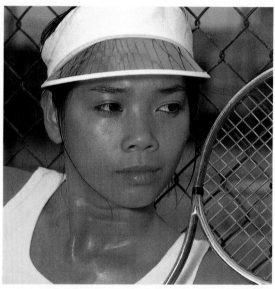

**BEFORE: Jade's personality is evident even without makeup. But color accents her beautiful features, and brings out her aura of power and sensuality.**

## WHAT TO USE

FOUNDATION: Alabaster Base mixed with White Toner
POWDER: Alabaster
CONTOUR: Under Cheekbone: Taupe; Jawline: Taupe; Nose: Taupe; Forehead: Taupe
CHEEKBONE: Pale Pink
EYES: Eyelid base: Pale Pink; Eye Contour: Taupe; Eyeliner: Black Liner over Charcoal Pencil; Eyelid: Inner Corner: Pale Pink; Outer Corner: Taupe
MASCARA: Black
EYEBROWS: Gray/Brown
LIP OUTLINE: Hot Pink Pencil
LIPSTICK: Shocking Pink
NAILS: Magenta Polish

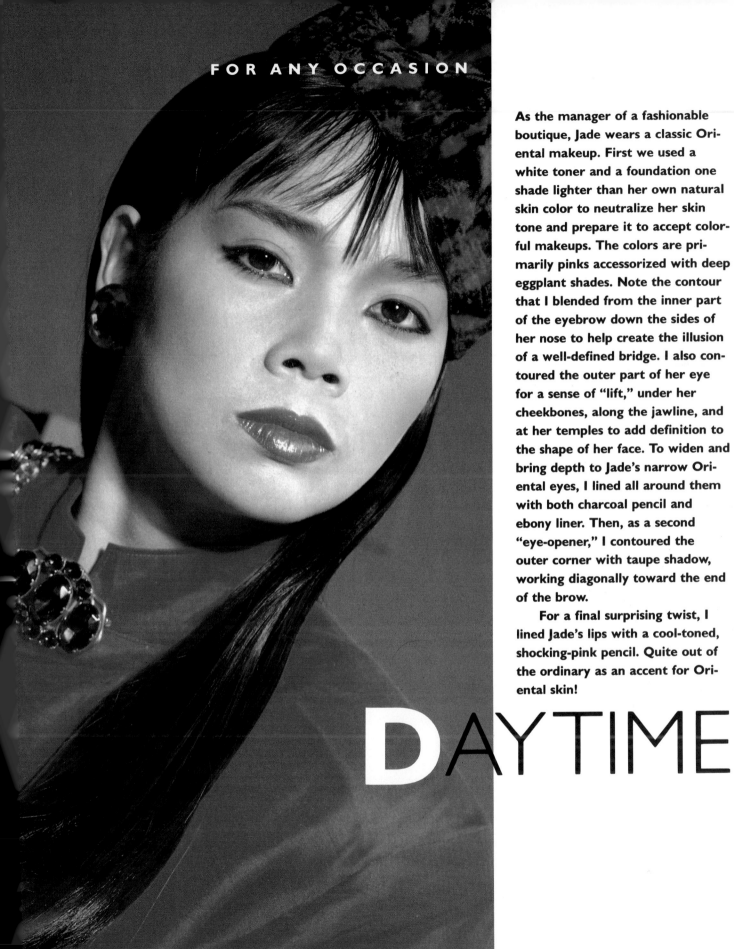

As the manager of a fashionable boutique, Jade wears a classic Oriental makeup. First we used a white toner and a foundation one shade lighter than her own natural skin color to neutralize her skin tone and prepare it to accept colorful makeups. The colors are primarily pinks accessorized with deep eggplant shades. Note the contour that I blended from the inner part of the eyebrow down the sides of her nose to help create the illusion of a well-defined bridge. I also contoured the outer part of her eye for a sense of "lift," under her cheekbones, along the jawline, and at her temples to add definition to the shape of her face. To widen and bring depth to Jade's narrow Oriental eyes, I lined all around them with both charcoal pencil and ebony liner. Then, as a second "eye-opener," I contoured the outer corner with taupe shadow, working diagonally toward the end of the brow.

For a final surprising twist, I lined Jade's lips with a cool-toned, shocking-pink pencil. Quite out of the ordinary as an accent for Oriental skin!

# DAYTIME

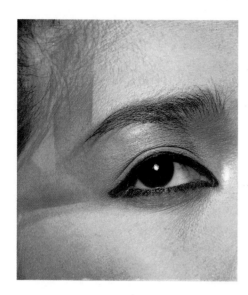

Again, Jade's skin tone is first primed with beige to help prepare it for color.

This warm, sophisticated, summery makeup look is composed primarily of oranges and other earth tones. Note, however, the wonderful effect of the two different color shadows—a cold fuchsia and a warm mango—over the outside of her eye. (To define the boundaries of these shadows beyond the lid, I used the card/airbrush technique described in the "Special Occasions, Special Effects" chapter of "The Makeup Lesson.") Alongside these compatible tones, the yellow-green shadow on the inner part of her lid is warm and sublime. And that colorful shadow sweep is elongated, accentuated by black liner...Altogether extraordinary eyes! Her lipstick is also in the orange family, and accessories match the colors of the makeup— green, mango, fuchsia, orange—for a double blast of Jade's exotic tropical heat.

## WHAT TO USE

FOUNDATION: Alabaster Base mixed with White Toner
POWDER: Alabaster
CONTOUR: Under Cheekbone: Light Brown; Jawline: Light Brown; Nose: Light Brown; Forehead: Light Brown
CHEEKBONE: Mango
EYES: Eyeliner: Black; Eyelid: Card/ Airbrush technique: Inner Corner— Peach/Sublime Lime, Outer Corner— Fuchsia/Mango
MASCARA: Black (lightly)
LIP OUTLINE: Orange Pencil
LIPSTICK: Rust
LIP HIGHLIGHT: Mango Shadow

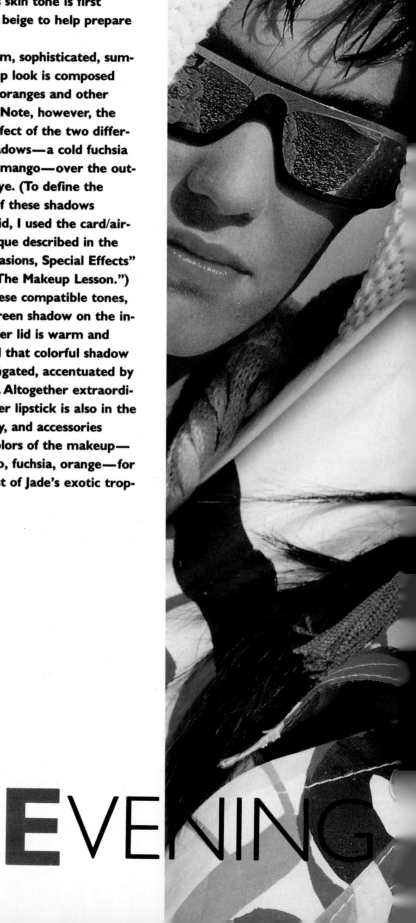

EVENING

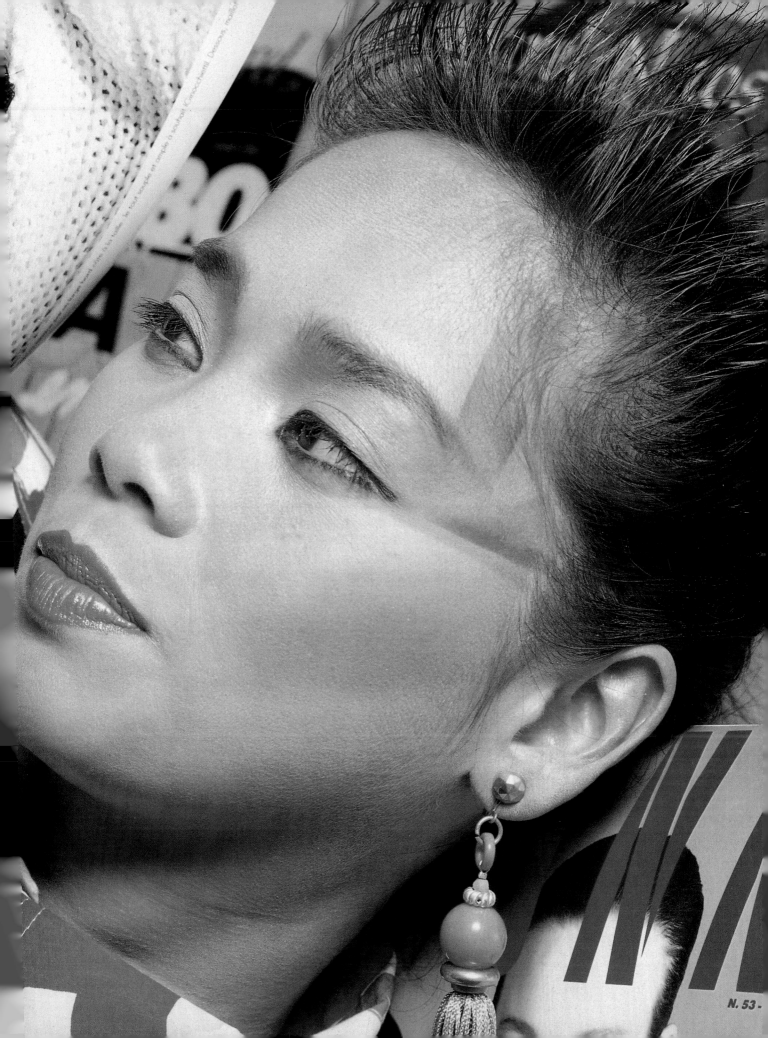

# NIGHTPLAY

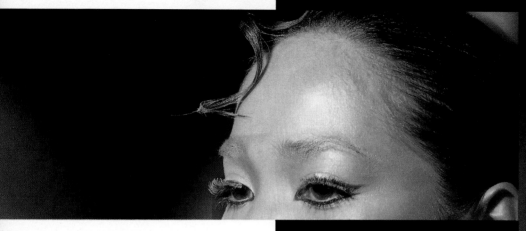

## SPECIAL EFFECTS

Here Jade truly breaks the color barrier. Because warm, yellow-toned skin contrasts with cold makeup colors, sometimes increasing sallowness, some experts have decreed that cold colors must never be used over naturally warm skin tones. But outdated rules are made to be broken...and that's exactly what we've done to spark up Jade's night on the town.

Jade's eyelashes, brows, lips, earrings are all touched with variations of cold silver. A translucent silver dust highlights her cheekbones; even the shadow color around her eyes is silver, blended with a widening accent of orchid at the outer corner. We've echoed the dazzling color scheme by lining Jade's inner rims in pewter pencil, then defined it all with a touch of black cake liner. The final touch—silver lashes. Sparkling!

To paint the town, Jade dressed in a black tuxedo, which is strikingly effective with her black hair. The unexpected interplay of her naturally warm skin color, the icy-cold makeup color scheme, and the stunning counterpoint of her clothing help Jade project an air of inner mystery and drama.

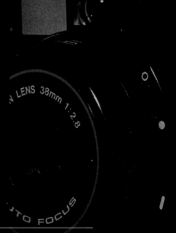

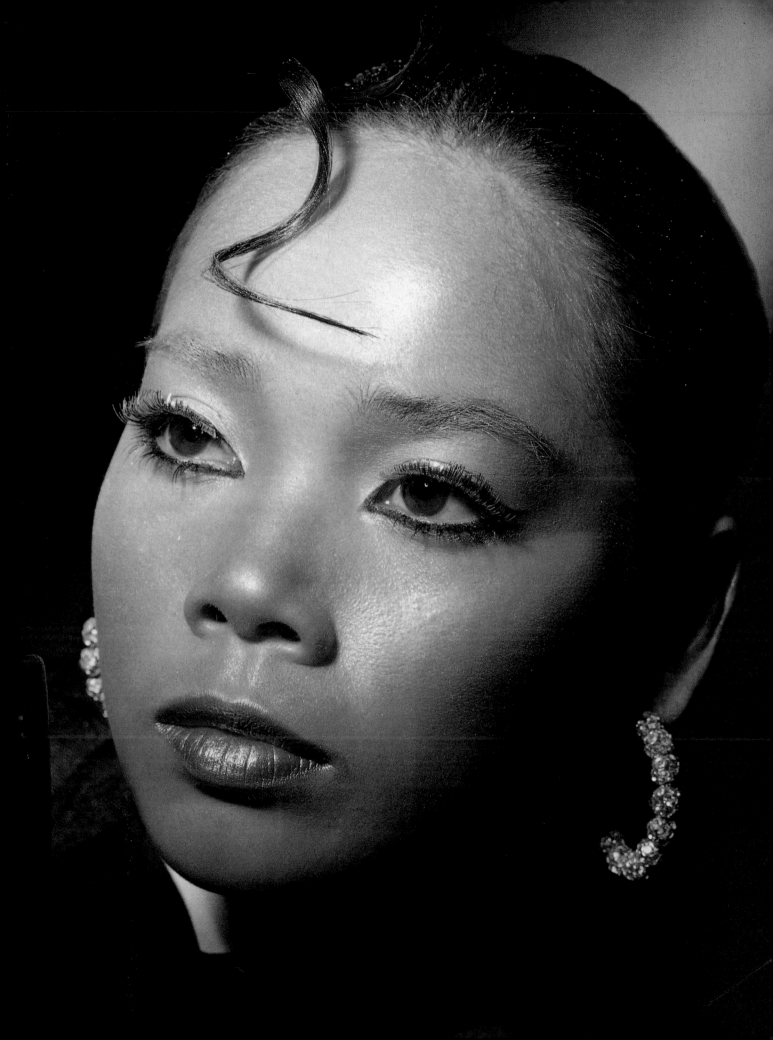

# THE HAPPY BRIDE

Debbie is our all-American girl, a platinum blonde with big, beautiful green eyes framed by bedroom lids and thick brows. Her nose is perfect, and her lips are lovely both in shape and color.

She's also very expressive, and we've chosen her to demonstrate the many moods of a bride. On her wedding day a bride glows as on no other day; she is . . . nervous . . . expectant . . . excited . . . blissful. She doesn't need strong colors to look sophisticated—but she does need special makeups to complement the spark that comes from inside on her special day.

Her makeover tones are delicately blended sheer browns, pinks, purples, and golds. Two of her looks are accented by extraordinary special effects; the other is so simple and pretty it would work for any occasion. Each of these makeups, as different as they are, is becoming and totally appropriate to the events of Debbie's day. Even with special effects, they are all simple in terms of color, ranging from uncluttered combinations of her basic colors to a makeup that's truly monochromatic. And Debbie, our bride, looks ravishing in every one.

**BEFORE: Young and pretty, nervous and expectant, Debbie drinks her morning tea. Her quicksilver moods will soon find expression in the total looks of a bride's day.**

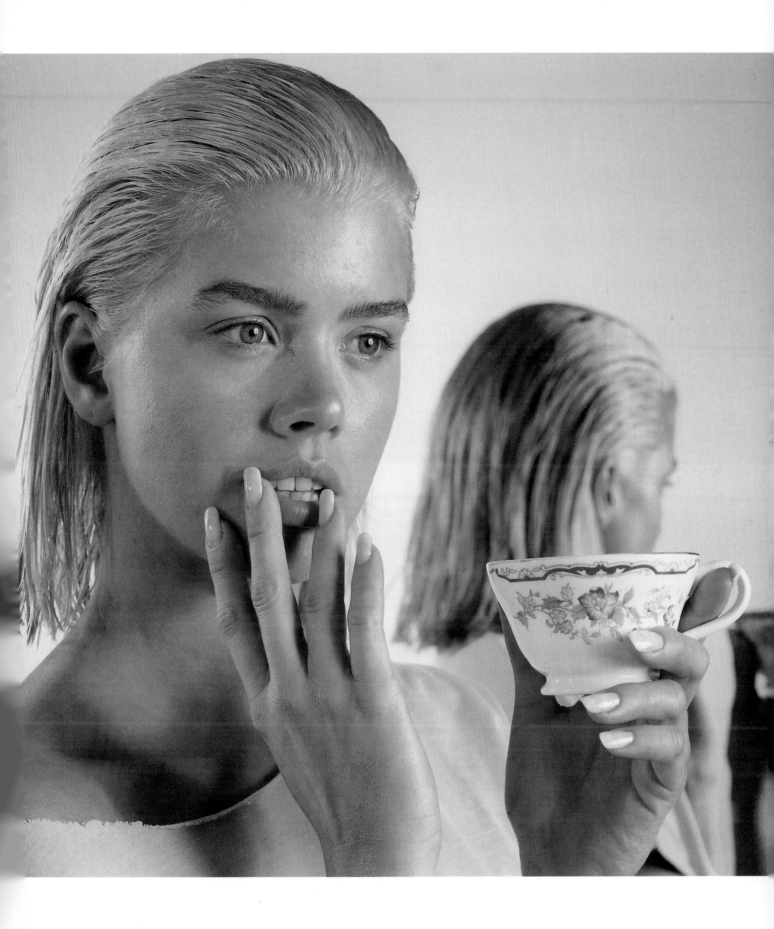

## FOR ANY OCCASION

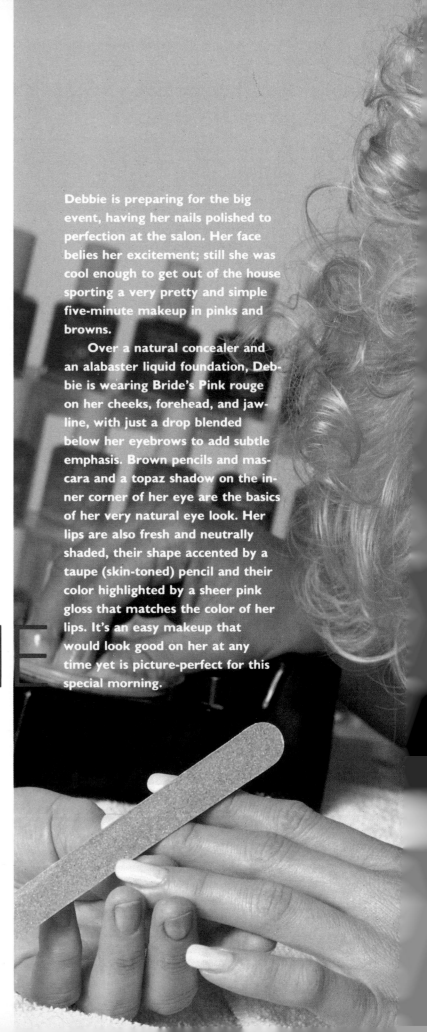

Debbie is preparing for the big event, having her nails polished to perfection at the salon. Her face belies her excitement; still she was cool enough to get out of the house sporting a very pretty and simple five-minute makeup in pinks and browns.

Over a natural concealer and an alabaster liquid foundation, Debbie is wearing Bride's Pink rouge on her cheeks, forehead, and jawline, with just a drop blended below her eyebrows to add subtle emphasis. Brown pencils and mascara and a topaz shadow on the inner corner of her eye are the basics of her very natural eye look. Her lips are also fresh and neutrally shaded, their shape accented by a taupe (skin-toned) pencil and their color highlighted by a sheer pink gloss that matches the color of her lips. It's an easy makeup that would look good on her at any time yet is picture-perfect for this special morning.

# DAYTIME

## WHAT TO USE

CONCEALER: Natural
FOUNDATION: Sheer Alabaster
Liquid Base
CONTOUR: Under Cheekbone: Bride's
Pink; Jawline: Bride's Pink; Forehead:
Bride's Pink
CHEEKBONE: Bride's Pink
EYES: Eyeliner: Coconut Pencil; Eyelid:
Inner Corner—Topaz Shadow, Outer
Corner—Espresso Pencil
MASCARA: Brown
BROW BONE: Bride's Pink
LIP OUTLINE: Taupe Pencil
LIP GLOSS: Hot Pink

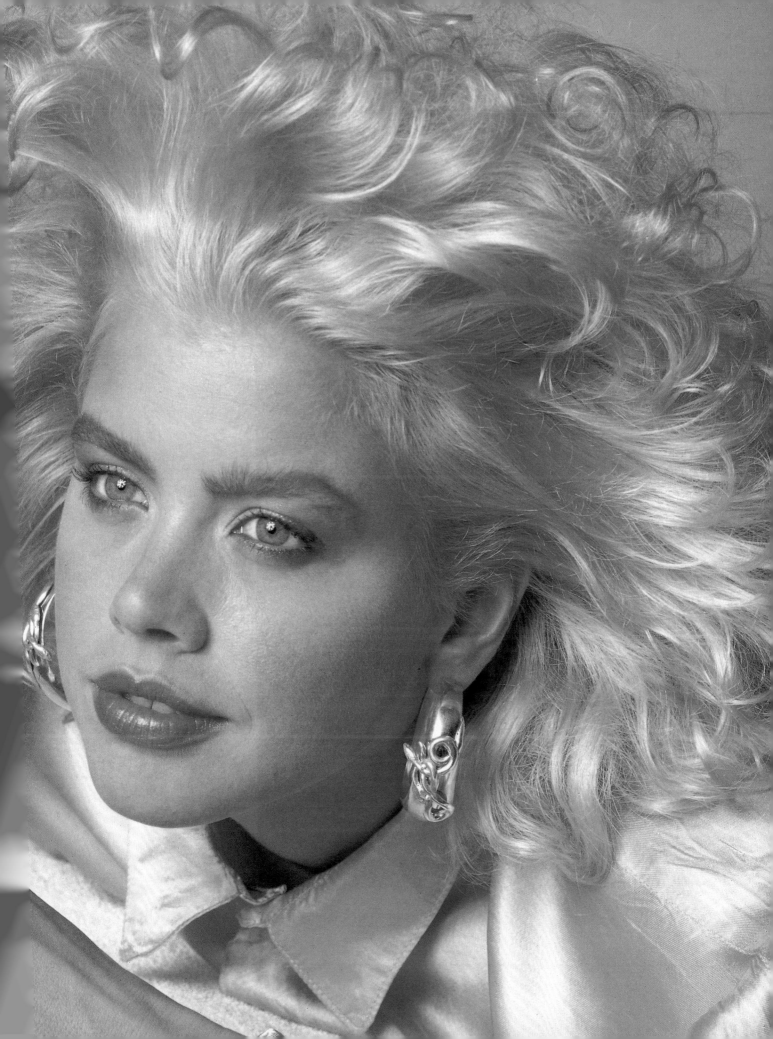

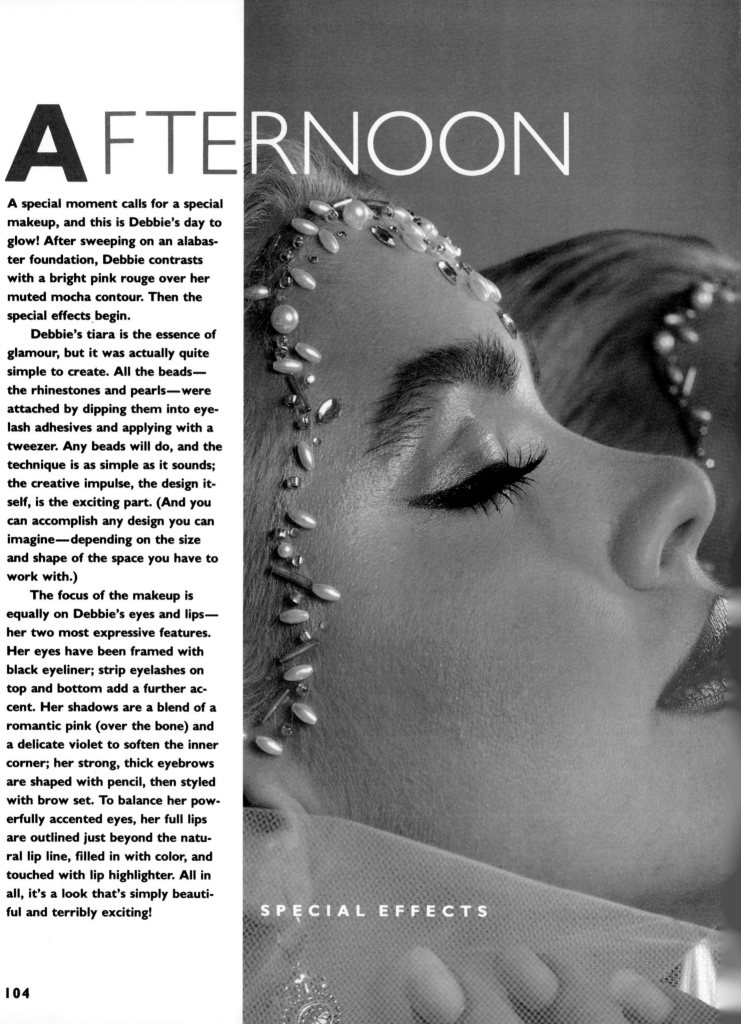

# **A**FTERNOON

A special moment calls for a special makeup, and this is Debbie's day to glow! After sweeping on an alabaster foundation, Debbie contrasts with a bright pink rouge over her muted mocha contour. Then the special effects begin.

Debbie's tiara is the essence of glamour, but it was actually quite simple to create. All the beads— the rhinestones and pearls—were attached by dipping them into eyelash adhesives and applying with a tweezer. Any beads will do, and the technique is as simple as it sounds; the creative impulse, the design itself, is the exciting part. (And you can accomplish any design you can imagine—depending on the size and shape of the space you have to work with.)

The focus of the makeup is equally on Debbie's eyes and lips— her two most expressive features. Her eyes have been framed with black eyeliner; strip eyelashes on top and bottom add a further accent. Her shadows are a blend of a romantic pink (over the bone) and a delicate violet to soften the inner corner; her strong, thick eyebrows are shaped with pencil, then styled with brow set. To balance her powerfully accented eyes, her full lips are outlined just beyond the natural lip line, filled in with color, and touched with lip highlighter. All in all, it's a look that's simply beautiful and terribly exciting!

SPECIAL EFFECTS

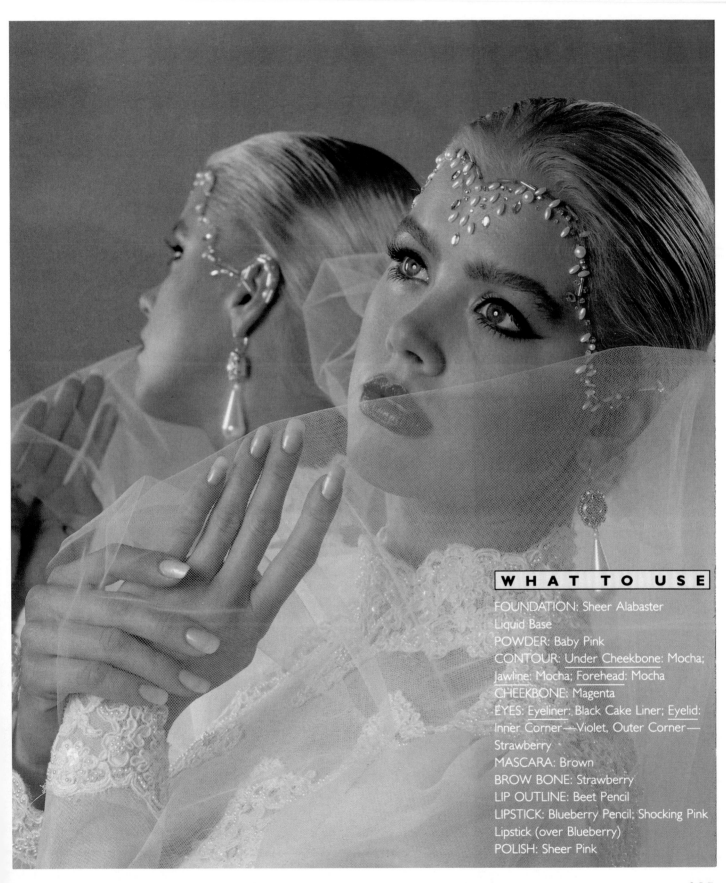

## W H A T  T O  U S E

FOUNDATION: Sheer Alabaster
Liquid Base
POWDER: Baby Pink
CONTOUR: Under Cheekbone: Mocha;
Jawline: Mocha; Forehead: Mocha
CHEEKBONE: Magenta
EYES: Eyeliner: Black Cake Liner; Eyelid:
Inner Corner—Violet, Outer Corner—
Strawberry
MASCARA: Brown
BROW BONE: Strawberry
LIP OUTLINE: Beet Pencil
LIPSTICK: Blueberry Pencil; Shocking Pink
Lipstick (over Blueberry)
POLISH: Sheer Pink

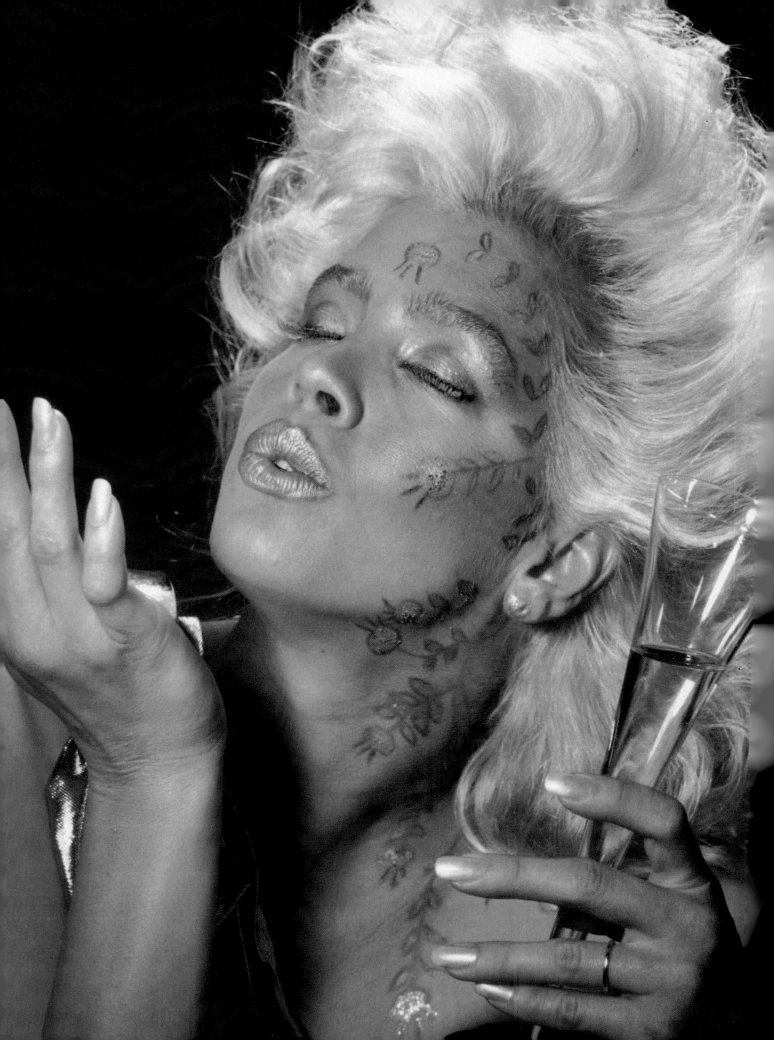

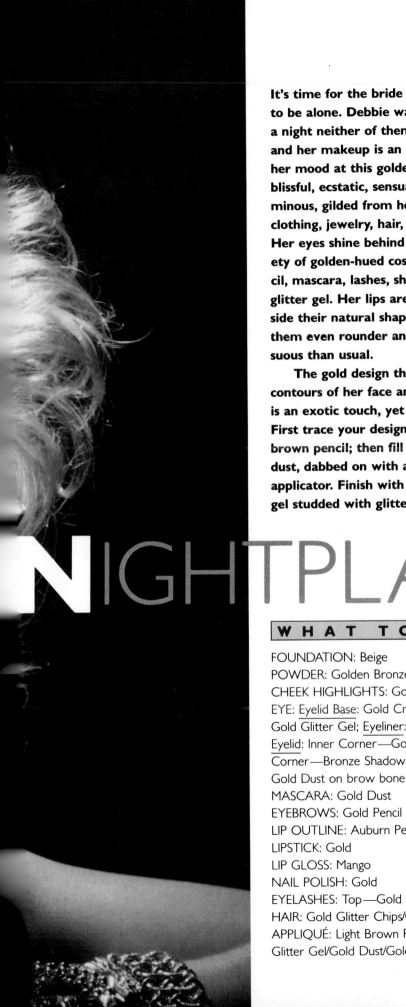

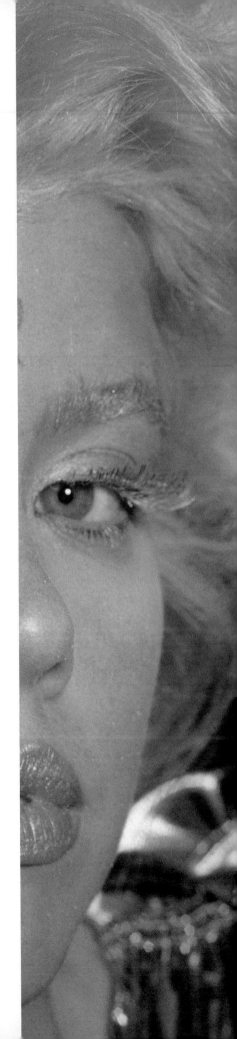

It's time for the bride and groom to be alone. Debbie wants it to be a night neither of them will forget, and her makeup is an expression of her mood at this golden moment: blissful, ecstatic, sensual. She is luminous, gilded from head to toe: clothing, jewelry, hair, and makeup. Her eyes shine behind a wide variety of golden-hued cosmetics: pencil, mascara, lashes, shadow, and glitter gel. Her lips are lined outside their natural shape, making them even rounder and more sensuous than usual.

The gold design that traces the contours of her face and shoulders is an exotic touch, yet easy to do: First trace your design with a thin brown pencil; then fill in with gold dust, dabbed on with a sponge-tip applicator. Finish with gold glitter gel studded with glitter chips.

# NIGHTPLAY

## WHAT TO USE

FOUNDATION: Beige
POWDER: Golden Bronze
CHEEK HIGHLIGHTS: Gold Dust
EYE: Eyelid Base: Gold Cream Shadow/
Gold Glitter Gel; Eyeliner: Gold Pencil;
Eyelid: Inner Corner—Gold Dust, Outer
Corner—Bronze Shadow; Eye Highlights:
Gold Dust on brow bone
MASCARA: Gold Dust
EYEBROWS: Gold Pencil
LIP OUTLINE: Auburn Pencil
LIPSTICK: Gold
LIP GLOSS: Mango
NAIL POLISH: Gold
EYELASHES: Top—Gold Strip Lashes
HAIR: Gold Glitter Chips/Gold Dust
APPLIQUÉ: Light Brown Pencil/Gold
Glitter Gel/Gold Dust/Gold Glitter Chips

# JENNIFER GATTI:
# YOUNG
# AND FASHIONABLE

Jennifer's youth, her beautiful dark auburn hair, big green eyes, strong features, and bone structure combine intensity with innocence.

She's a sporty outdoor type, but at times she wants to look elegant, sophisticated, and mature. How can we transform her look? With her wide forehead and pronounced bone structure her face allows for many possibilities of contour and shading: her deep-green eyes easily accept either a warm or a cold frame.

Her skin, however, is delicate, sensitive, and thin, giving her a naturally cold skin tone—transparent and reddish from broken capillaries near the skin surface. Some experts contend that women with Jennifer's skin tone should only wear makeup colors that warm up their coloration, but that's terribly limiting for such an active young woman. Watch her looks run the gamut from a sheer transparent five-minute look and a warm, sophisticated evening look—both in her basic colors—to a silvery nightplay makeup that breaks Jennifer's color barrier and adds an aura of elegance and mystery to her glowing youth.

**BEFORE: Jennifer is young and lovely, and her face combines innocence with strength of character. She's a complex individual who wants her uniqueness to show.**

108

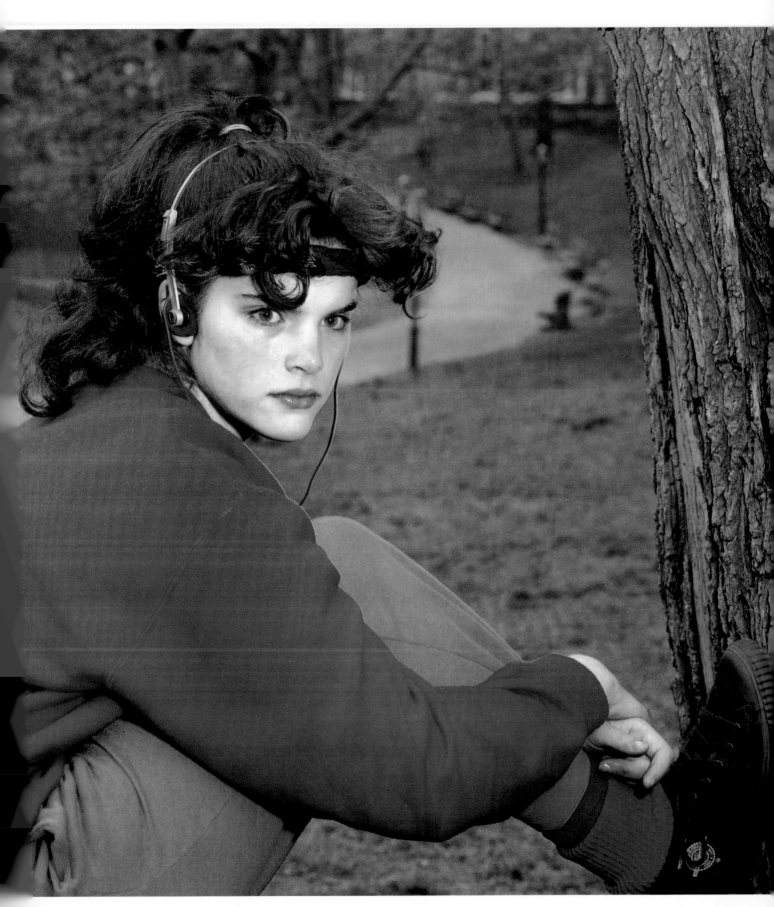

Here Jennifer wears a fast and easy five-minute makeup that shows her to be a self-assured young woman who's comfortable on the ladder to success without hiding her sensuality. After dusting on a sheer pressed powder instead of foundation, Jennifer applies makeup colors—khakis and wine tones—that complement her dark auburn hair and green eyes no matter what the occasion. The browns of the makeup neutralize the redness in her skin. Contour on the sides of her nose narrows it, while above her eyebrows it deemphasizes the bone; her lips are stained (by applying lipstick and blotting with a tissue) in a natural color. The final effect—warm and fresh.

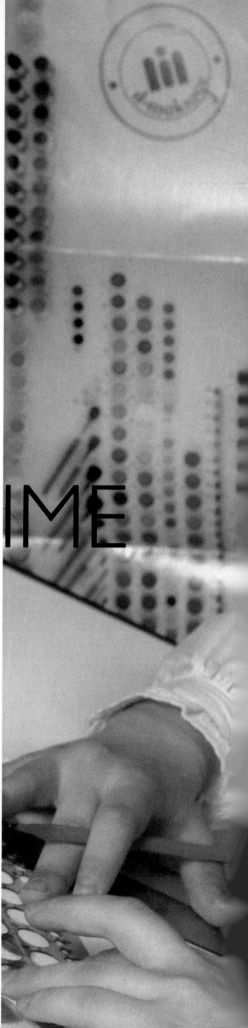

FOR ANY OCCASION 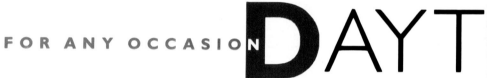DAYTIME

## WHAT TO USE

FOUNDATION: Alabaster Pressed Powder
CONTOUR: Under Cheekbone: Light Brown; Jawline: Light Brown; Nose: Light Brown; Forehead: Light Brown
CHEEKBONE: Bordeaux
EYES: Eye Contour: Khaki Shadow; Eyelid: Inner Corner—Strawberry Shadow, Outer Corner—Khaki Shadow
MASCARA: Black
EYEBROWS: Brow Set
LIP OUTLINE: Beet Pencil
LIPSTICK: Brown Velvet

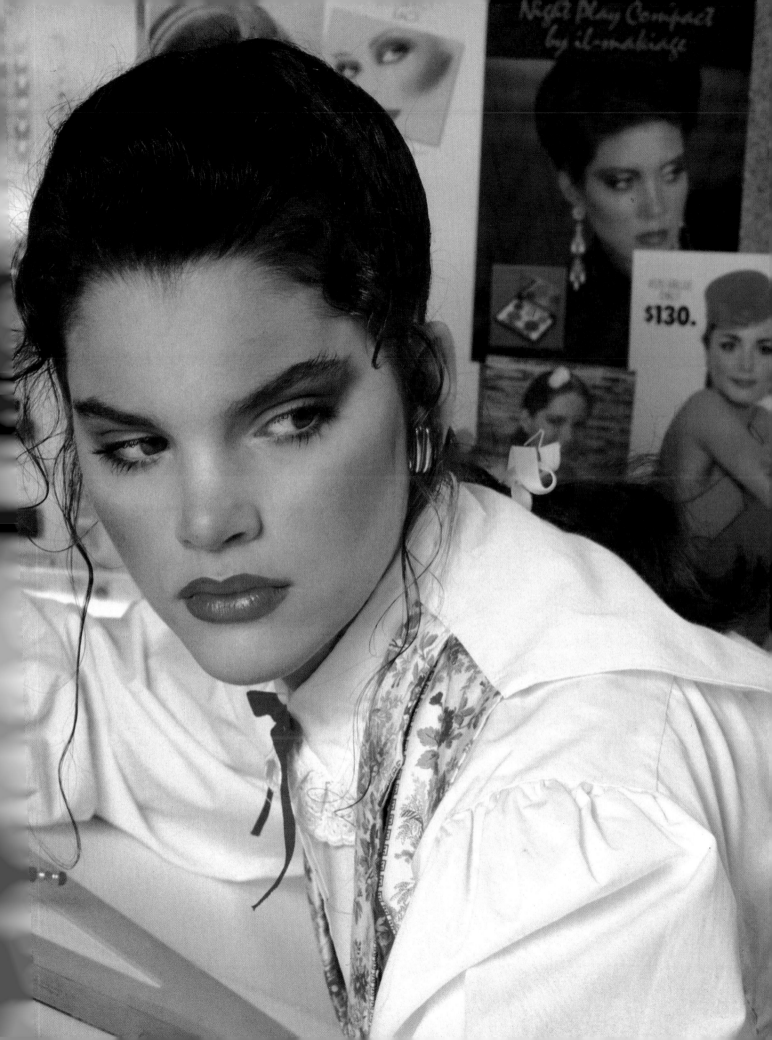

After work, Jennifer is made up in minutes for her dinner date—with a sophisticated evening look applied directly over her five-minute office makeup. Again we've used deep, rich browns to bring out Jennifer's beauty, but with splashes of yellow and gold to make it even warmer than her daytime look. In place of lipstick she wears a khaki shadow dramatically topped with a sheer red lip gloss. A dusting of mustard-colored translucent powder adds a final touch of color. It's a warm makeup designed to reflect the colors of autumn, and it's excellent for all occasions that require a little sophistication.

# EVENING
### A LITTLE SOPHISTICATION

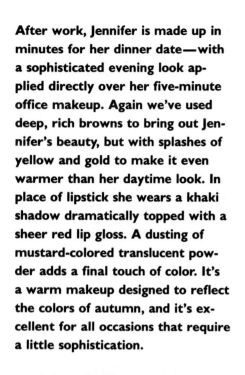

## WHAT TO USE

FOUNDATION: Alabaster Pressed Powder
CONTOUR: Under Cheekbone: Light Brown; Jawline: Light Brown; Nose: Light Brown; Forehead: Light Brown
CHEEKBONE: Raisin
CHEEKBONE HIGHLIGHTS: Mustard Shadow
EYES: Eye Contour: Khaki Shadow; Eyelid: Inner Corner—Brass Dust, Outer Corner—Khaki Shadow; Eye Highlights: Gold Cream Shadow over brow bone
MASCARA: Black
LIP OUTLINE: Auburn Pencil
FINISH: Yellow Transparent Powder

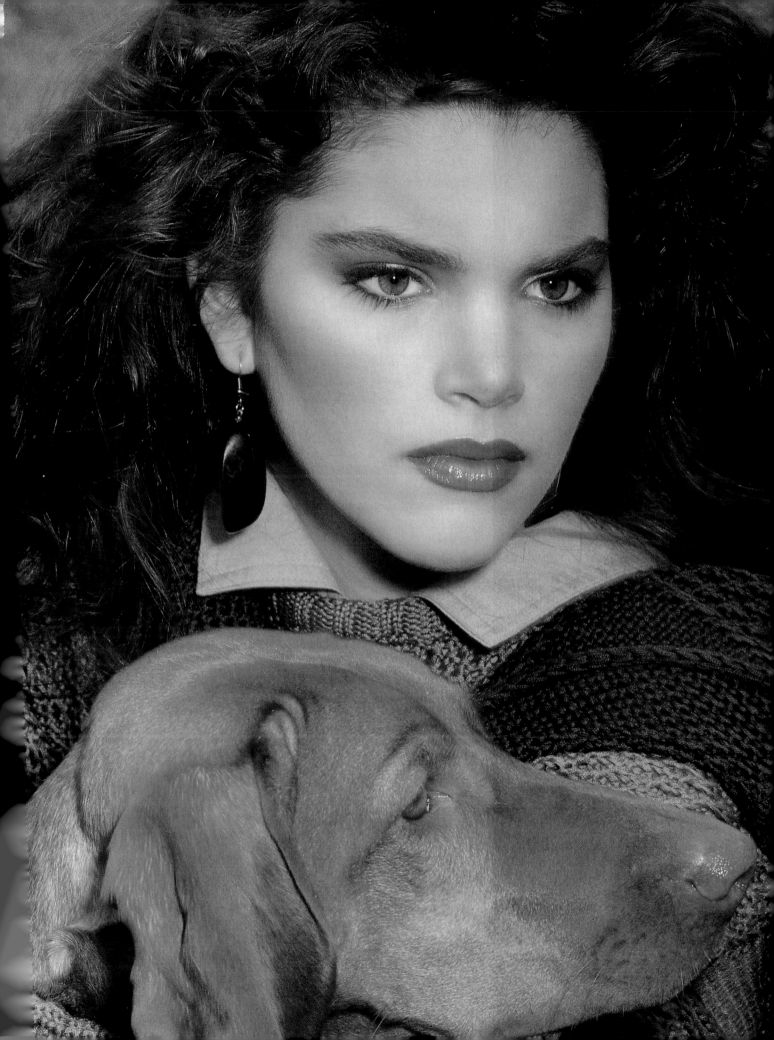

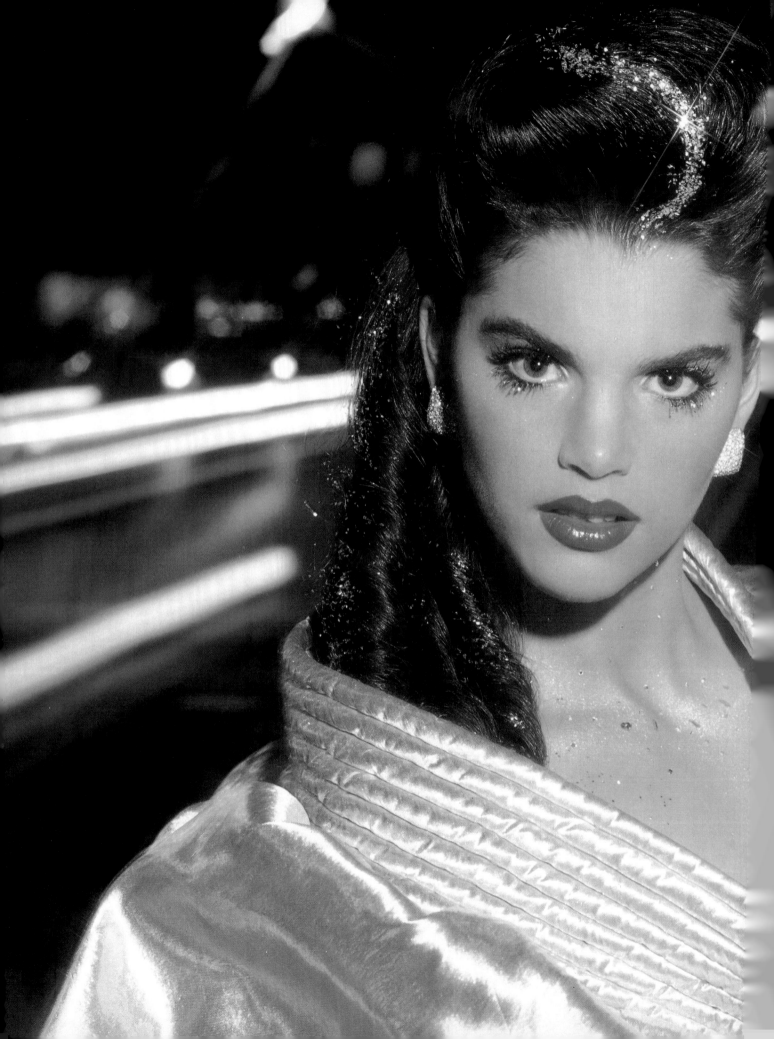

Jennifer breaks the color barrier with a glittery nightplay look. Her lids and lower lashes are highlighted in blue; a bright shadow extended upward and diagonally to widen her beautiful eyes. And she sparkles in silver—on her lashes, in her hair, on her neck and shoulders. Even her individual false eyelashes, applied on outer corners both top and bottom, have been tipped in silver glitter. (To apply your own nightplay magic, dip lash tips in moisturizer, then touch with glitter dust.) The silver shine that accents her neckline as well as her hair can all be washed off: The glittering bits are sprinkled into the hair right after it's sprayed; eyelash glue and tweezers are used to apply the silver sparkle to her neckline. It's a look that's dominated by cold colors, but the addition of warm reddish-orange lipstick softens and warms it. The result? Even on a cold winter night, Jennifer radiates plenty of sophisticated heat.

## SPECIAL EFFECTS

# NIGHTPLAY

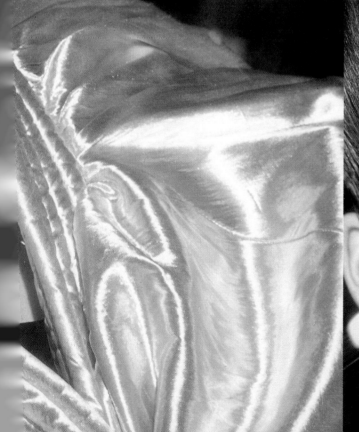

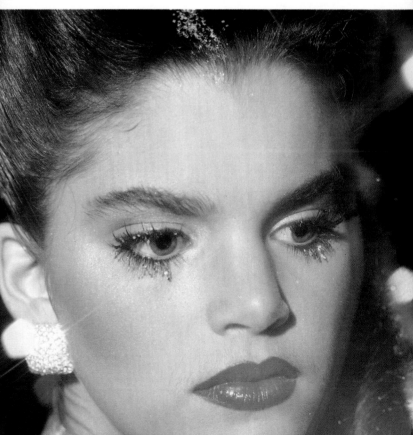

# ZACKI MURPHY:

# WOMAN PRESIDENT

Zacki is a working professional, a mother, and a mature woman who must somehow find the time for everything, Still, her expressive eyes and lovely lips glow with a wonderful, easy smile.

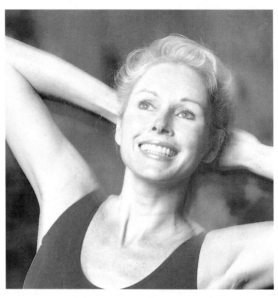

Some women think heavy makeups will compensate for dry skin lines, and diminish the creases that come with maturity.

Not so! Zacki takes proper care of her pretty skin, which means moisturizing and keeping makeup to a minimum. That's how dry skin lines are really eliminated.

Here she wears a natural-looking makeup for the office, very soft vacation makeup appropriate for a quick, revitalizing trip, and a shimmering evening makeup that incorporates some startling special effects. We worked within a range of her basic colors; varying techniques of application to suit the time and the place.

We also highlighted her hair with a henna rinse; a champagne or gold henna rinse or gel turns gray into ash highlights and can be washed out in your next shampoo. For more permanent coloring, a single-process henna pack (see step-by-step instructions in the "Healthy Hair" chapter of "Beauty Basics") will add highlights for two or three months; a double process will cover the gray completely.

**BEFORE: Zacki makes sure to leave enough time in her busy schedule to work off stress and keep in shape. She leads a full life and expresses it in her makeups.**

## WHAT TO USE

FOUNDATION: Beige
CONTOUR: Under Cheekbones: Light Brown; Jawline: Light Brown
CHEEKBONE: Cantaloupe
CHEEKBONE HIGHLIGHTS: Ivory Shadow
EYES: Eye Contour: Wood; Eyeliner: Coconut Pencil; Eyelid Base: Cantaloupe Shadow; Eye Highlights: Cantaloupe on brow bone
LIP OUTLINE: Auburn Pencil
LIPSTICK: Peach
NAIL POLISH: Nude

116

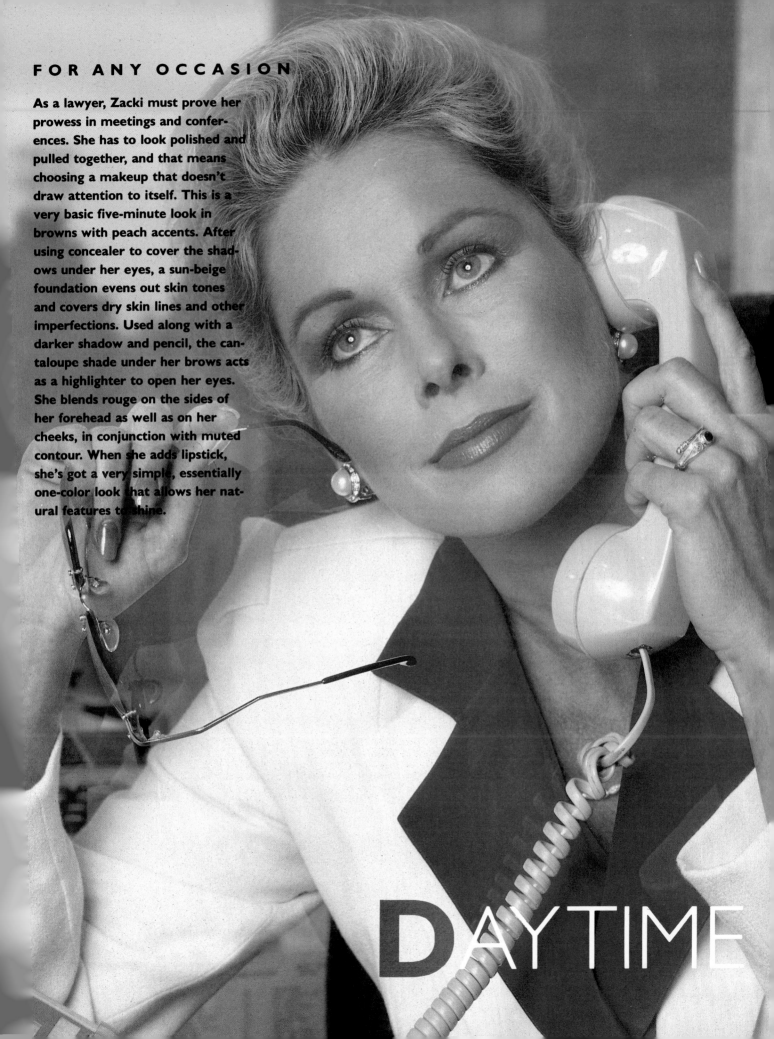

## FOR ANY OCCASION

As a lawyer, Zacki must prove her prowess in meetings and conferences. She has to look polished and pulled together, and that means choosing a makeup that doesn't draw attention to itself. This is a very basic five-minute look in browns with peach accents. After using concealer to cover the shadows under her eyes, a sun-beige foundation evens out skin tones and covers dry skin lines and other imperfections. Used along with a darker shadow and pencil, the cantaloupe shade under her brows acts as a highlighter to open her eyes. She blends rouge on the sides of her forehead as well as on her cheeks, in conjunction with muted contour. When she adds lipstick, she's got a very simple, essentially one-color look that allows her natural features to shine.

# DAYTIME

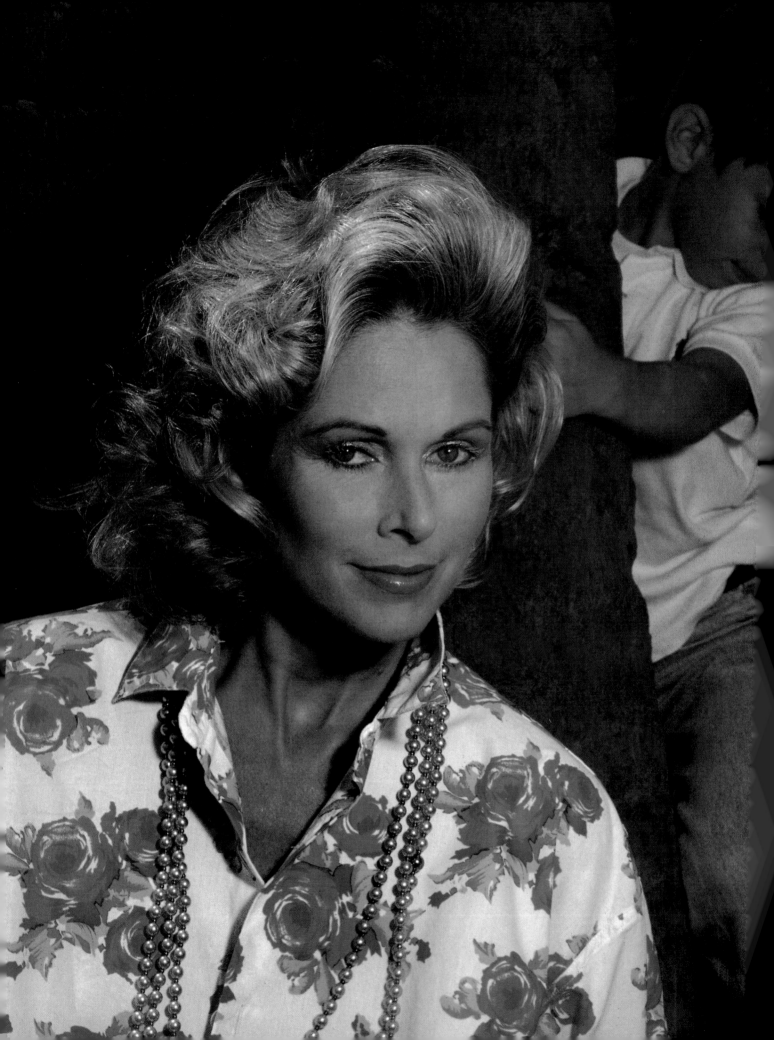

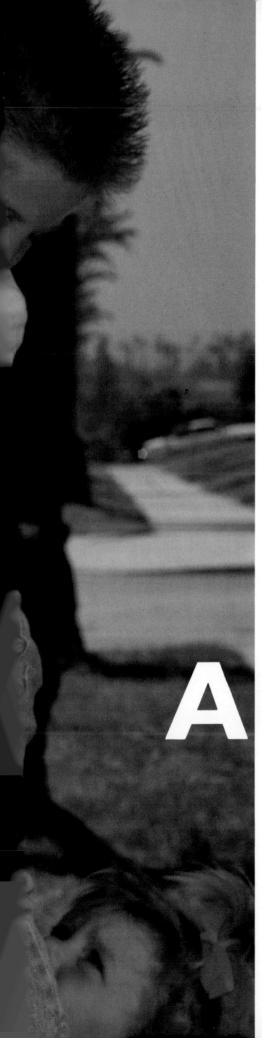

## REST AND RELAXATION

Here's a daytime resort makeup that's both attractive and protective of Zacki's skin. It starts with a sunscreen instead of a moisturizer. (Although a more mature woman is further protected by putting a foundation-based makeup over her sunscreen, *everyone* should *always* wear sunscreen at the beach, with makeup or without.) Next, transparent powder is dabbed over the T-zone, where most women, even those with dry skin, tend to get a little shiny. Her rouge adds a healthy brownish red glow to Zacki's cheeks, and no contour is used. The blue and green combination around her eyes helps bring out their color. And the sheer red gloss outlined with red pencil not only adds color to her lips but moisturizes them as well. It's a five-minute makeup that truly protects...colorfully.

# AFTERNOON

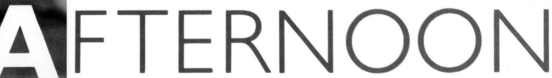

**WHAT TO USE**

FOUNDATION: Sunscreen; Beige Liquid Base
POWDER: Beige
CHEEKBONE: Cognac
EYES: <u>Eyelid</u>: Inner Corner—Gold Dust, Outer Corner—Bright Blue; <u>Eye Highlights</u>: Beige on brow bone
<u>Eyeliner</u>: Coconut pencil (optional)
MASCARA: Blue
EYEBROWS: Taupe Pencil
LIP OUTLINE: Red Pencil
LIP GLOSS: Sheer Red

# NIGHT

Zacki is the essence of mature glamour as she attends a gala benefit at the opera in a makeup that incorporates subtle flashes of iridescence (in the only places a woman past her early thirties should ever wear it).

First, a rouge is blended down from her cheekbone as a contour; then a pink rouge is blended up over an iridescent cream highlighter added on top of the bone to further accentuate it. Her eyes are shaped and shaded with color. A dark eggplant shadow in the crease "lifts" the eye; a grayish-brown shadow at the outer edge elongates it. Zacki's eggplant eyeliner, the same powder shadow used on her lids, is applied as close as possible to the lashes. She's also wearing blue mascara, along with brown strip eyelashes on top and bottom and two or three individual lashes on the outer corner of each eye to further accentuate and open it. A very pale pink iridescent highlighter is dusted below her brows and on her lower lid.

Her colorful lip makeup is sure to last all night: First, foundation is blended over lips, then lips are dusted with transparent powder. A lip line of concealer is drawn above the real lip line to accent lip shape. Lips are then outlined with pencil, filled in with lipstick, and outline and lipstick are blended. The finishing touch is a pink highlighter on the center of the lips.

It's a balanced makeup that uses just enough iridescence to make Zacki's night at the opera an occasion of sparkling sophistication.

## WHAT TO USE

FOUNDATION: Beige Liquid Base
POWDER: Beige
CHEEKBONE: Pale Pink
CHEEKBONE HIGHLIGHTS: Silver Cream Highlighter
EYES: Eyelid Base: Pink Dust; Eye Contour: Eggplant Shadow; Eyeliner: Eggplant Pencil with Black Liner over it; Eyelid: Inner Corner—Pink Dust, Outer Corner—Gray/Brown Shadow; Eye Highlights: Pink Dust on brow bone
MASCARA: Blue
EYEBROWS: Taupe Pencil
LIP OUTLINE: Hot Pink Pencil
LIPSTICK: Shocking Pink
LIP HIGHLIGHT: Pink Dust
EYELASHES: Top—Strip; Bottom—Strip; Outer Corners—2–3 individual lashes

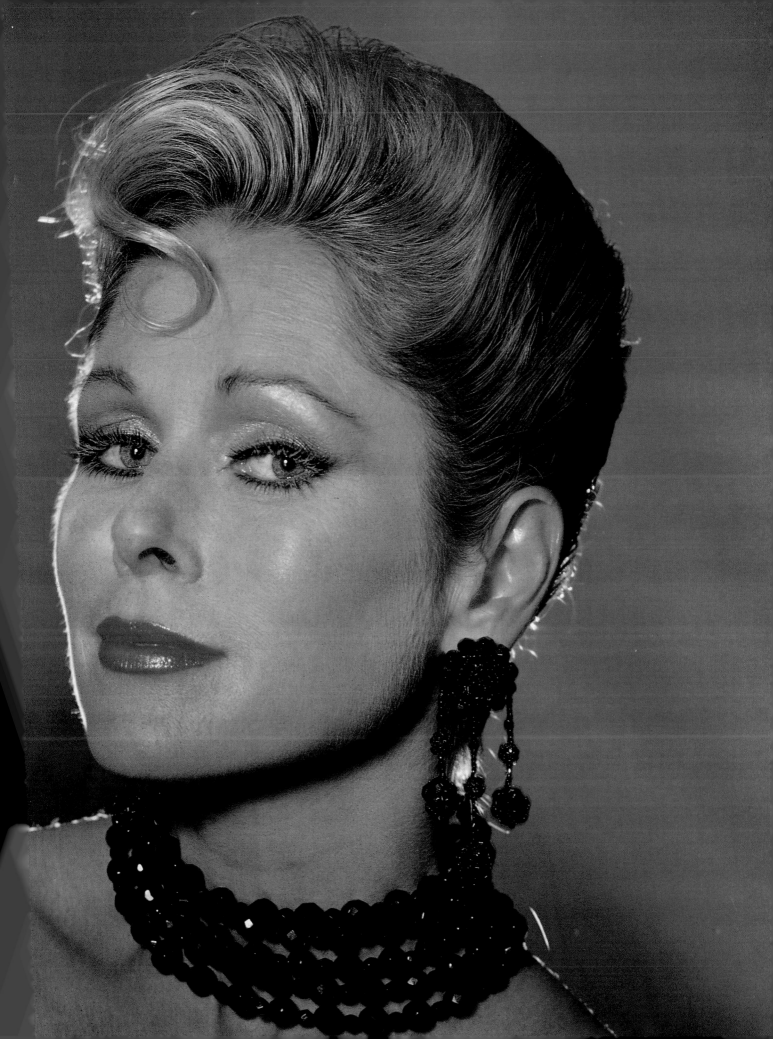

# LISA HEWITT:

# LOVE ME TENDER

Lisa's natural sensitivity finds its expression in her beautiful, round blue-gray eyes (and a wide-open lid space with which to emphasize them), lovely lips, classic oval-shaped face, and fine features.

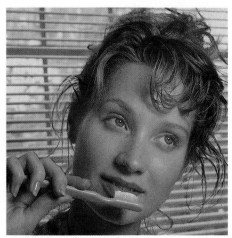

She also has a redhead's very fair skin and freckles. Women with this coloring often feel limited to oranges and reddish-browns when choosing makeup colors, but there is no reason why a woman with looks like Lisa's—or yours—can't break the color barrier. Indeed, one of the makeups I chose for her is based on pink, a color you might have thought impossible for a redhead. And as for her eyes, it's no illusion: Lisa's really do change color from green to blue in these photos when enhanced by makeup accessories.

Despite her naturally soft and sensitive looks, Lisa, like all women, has many moods. In these makeup transformations she expresses some of them, from delicate and demure to wild and adventurous to reserved and self-assured.

**BEFORE: Don't let Lisa's freckles, wide-open eyes, and delicate features deceive you; she's really a woman who can be whoever she wants to be.**

## WHAT TO USE

CONCEALER: Natural
FOUNDATION: Alabaster
POWDER: Alabaster
CONTOUR: Under Cheekbone: Light Brown; Jawline: Light Brown; Nose: Light Brown; Forehead: Light Brown
CHEEKBONE: Pale Pink
EYES: Eyelid Base: Pale Pink; Eye Contour: China Blue; Eyelid: Inner Corner—Rose, Outer Corner—China Blue; Eye Highlights: Pale Pink Iridescent Shadow on brow bone
MASCARA: Blue
EYEBROWS: Taupe Pencil
LIP OUTLINE: Soft Pink Pencil
LIP GLOSS: Pink
NAILS: Magenta

122

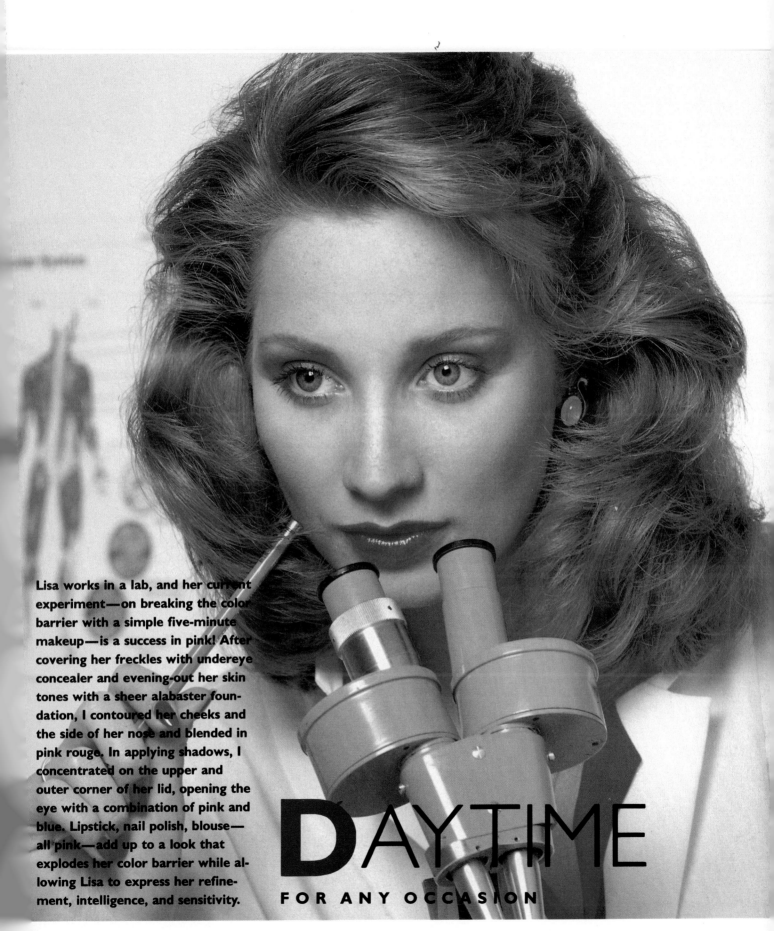

Lisa works in a lab, and her current experiment—on breaking the color barrier with a simple five-minute makeup—is a success in pink! After covering her freckles with undereye concealer and evening-out her skin tones with a sheer alabaster foundation, I contoured her cheeks and the side of her nose and blended in pink rouge. In applying shadows, I concentrated on the upper and outer corner of her lid, opening the eye with a combination of pink and blue. Lipstick, nail polish, blouse—all pink—add up to a look that explodes her color barrier while allowing Lisa to express her refinement, intelligence, and sensitivity.

# DAYTIME
## FOR ANY OCCASION

## A LITTLE SOPHISTICATION

Lisa's on safari: She's still the same vulnerable girl, but out in the bush she feels like letting go a bit and allowing her own wild side to come through. Here she captures the earthy tones of the environment with a makeup and accessories that accent her own natural coloration. Some instant color (in the form of henna gel) combed into her hair brings out its natural red highlights; an auburn pencil on her brows echoes that accent; and blue/green shadows accentuate the green in her eyes. Brown-wine lips, sun-bronze colored powder, and brown outfit finish the look—wild and natural in basic shades of green and brown.

# AFTERNOON

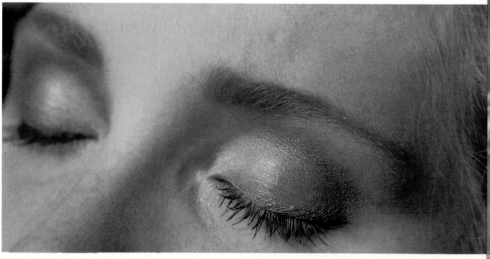

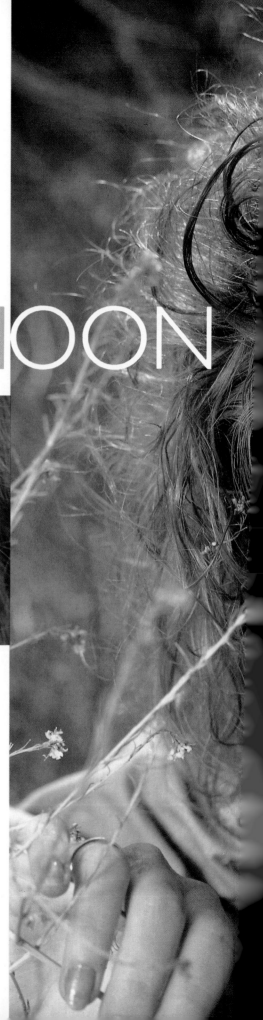

### WHAT TO USE

FOUNDATION: Sunny Beige Liquid Base
POWDER: Bronze
CONTOUR: Under Cheekbone: Light Brown; Jawline: Light Brown; Nose: Light Brown; Forehead: Light Brown
CHEEKBONE: Mocha
EYES: Eyelid Base: Sand Shadow; Eye Contour: Forest Green (in geometric pattern); Eyeliner: Kohl Green Pencil inside eye; Eye Highlights: Sand Shadow on brow bone
MASCARA: Brown
EYEBROWS: Light Brown Shadow
LIP OUTLINE: Auburn Pencil
LIPSTICK: Cognac
NAILS: Nude Polish

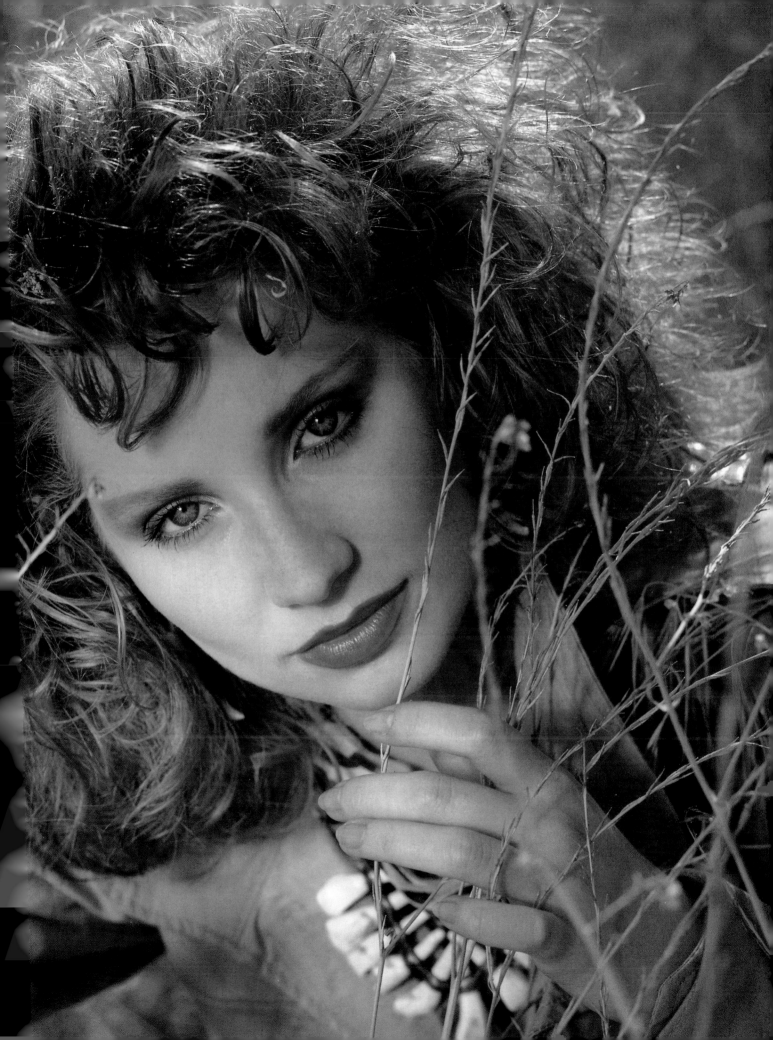

In her afternoon safari makeup Lisa blended into her environment; here at a garden party she stands in vivid contrast. It's a very sophisticated look, and the woman who wears it is obviously completely self-assured.

Much of the effect comes from accenting the classic shape of her face: Lisa's hair is up and off her forehead; her jawline, her cheeks, the cleft of her chin, the sides of her forehead are all contoured to create an even more impressively balanced oval; her nose is narrowed; her eyelids are wide and clean, and her eyebrows are brushed. Black kohl drawn inside the rim of her eye, black eyeliner, and sparse top and bottom strip eyelashes accentuate her eyes, now seemingly deep blue in contrast to the vivid greens of the garden. It's a total look achieved by the careful coordination of related colors: an orange silk blouse perfectly matched to lips; yellow and orange shadows; a beige finishing powder. It all adds up to a woman who looks refined, reserved, and marvelously put-together.

# NIGHTPLAY

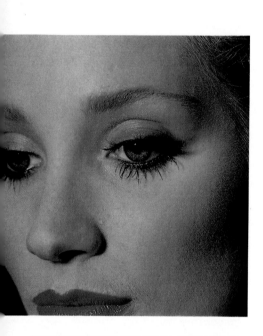

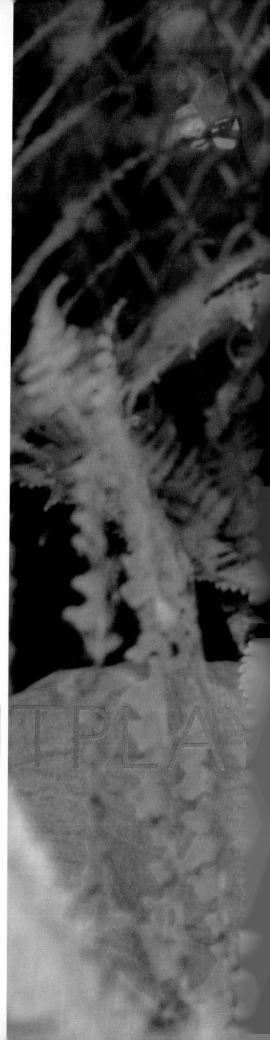

## WHAT TO USE

FOUNDATION: Sunny Beige Liquid Base
POWDER: Alabaster
CONTOUR: Under Cheekbone: Light Brown; Jawline: Light Brown; Nose: Light Brown; Forehead: Light Brown
CHEEKBONE: Apricot
EYES: Eyeliner: Black Pencil inside eye; Eyelid: Inner Corner—Gilt and Apricot Shadows blended; Outer Corner—Black Pencil
Eye Highlights: Gilt Shadow
MASCARA: Black
EYEBROWS: Gilt Shadow
LIP OUTLINE: Orange Pencil
LIPSTICK: Bright Orange

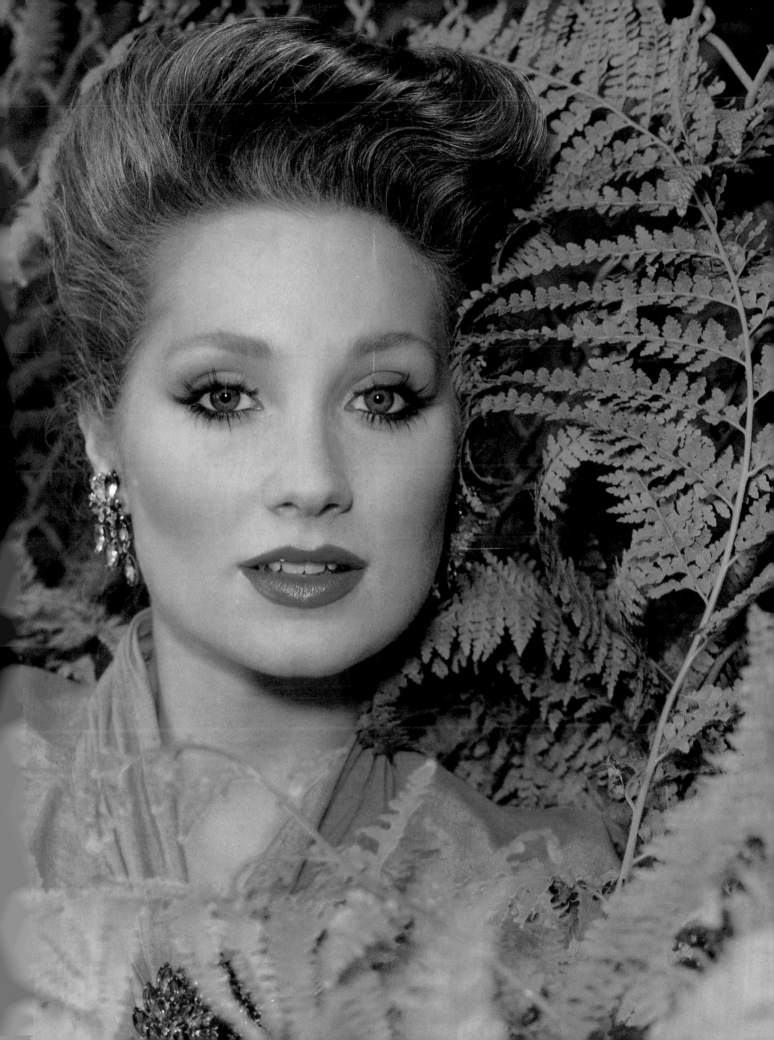

# VIBRANT AND VERSATILE

Kersti is a lovely young black woman with a *café au lait* complexion and naturally light brown hair that gets even lighter in the sun. The keys to her unique beauty are her alluring eyes, brows, and lips.

There are many sides to Kersti's personality: At times she is serious and contemplative, at others spontaneous and fun-loving; she is sophisticated, yet she relishes those occasions when she can be totally outrageous. And she sees no contradiction in any part of her lifestyle.

Kersti wants makeup to fit her every mood. Here we've given her a very modest five-minute look, a festive "feel good" makeup, and a daring, wild special effects look. She's beautiful—and different—in each.

In doing Kersti's makeups I concentrated on a basic beauty principle: Accentuate your best and no one will notice that you're not perfect. (And of course *no one* is.) Like most of us, Kersti's complexion shows variations in skin tone, and other small imperfections. I used a good foundation to even out her skin, then moved on from there to highlight those features that make her beautiful.

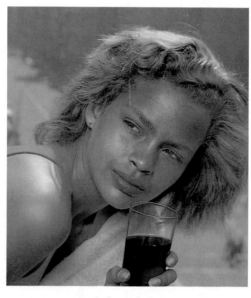

**BEFORE: Kersti is a healthy, active, modern young woman with varied interests and activities. Makeup helps bring out her best—whatever mood she's in.**

## WHAT TO USE

FOUNDATION: Bronze Liquid Base
POWDER: Peach
CHEEKBONE: Blueberry Pencil
EYES: Eye Contour: Blueberry Pencil; Eyeliner: Blueberry Pencil; Eyelid: Inner Corner—Mocha Shadow, Outer Corner—Khaki Shadow
MASCARA: Brown
LIP OUTLINE: Blueberry Pencil
LIP GLOSS: Clear

Kersti is tuning up before an audition. A good first impression is important, both in the way she sounds and in the way she looks. Since last-minute open calls make it necessary for Kersti to get out of the house fast, she wanted a five-minute makeup that was both unique and pretty. Here her healthy glow comes from her plum-toned makeup with sheer accents. Her most beautiful features—her eyes, lips, cheekbones—are all highlighted in compatible makeup colors—blueberry, khaki, and mocha—and brown mascara brings a further soft emphasis to her eyes. (When hair and makeup colors are not black, I generally stay away from black mascara for a daytime look.) It's all very natural looking, simple—and in tune with Kersti's busy life.

# DAYTIME

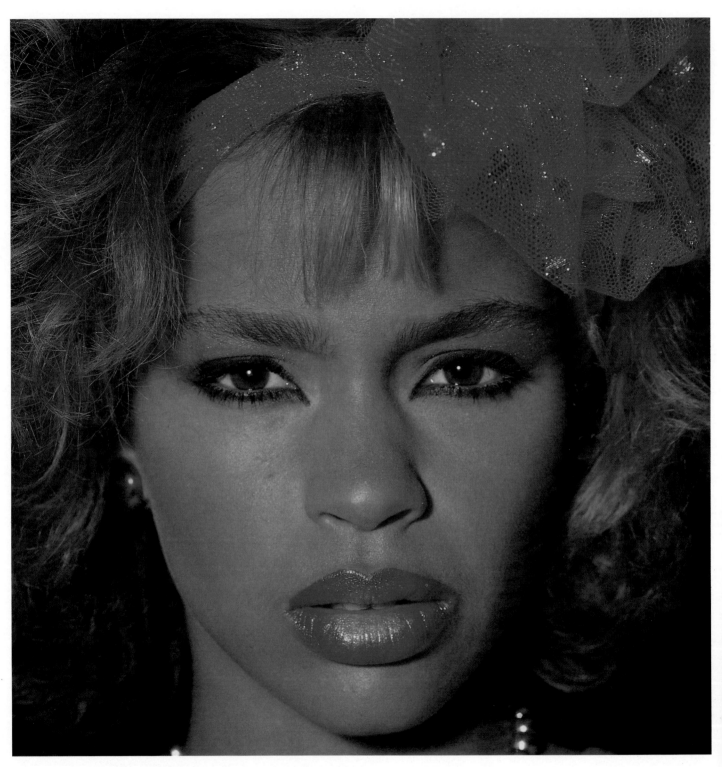

A LITTLE SOPHISTICATION

Kersti wants to have a good time on her birthday, and an extra special, festive, and outright sexy makeup is just the thing for her party. This is a makeup that breaks the color barrier with aplomb—bright red accents light up skin tones that supposedly can't warm up to red. The shapes of both her eyes and lips are emphasized: eyes with aquamarine kohl inside the rim and black eyeliner all around, lips with a gold gloss accent in the center of the lower lip and an upward extension of the natural line of the upper lip. Brass-colored dust highlights Kersti's eyelids, and a combination of sun-bronze and pink powder adds a finishing touch to her cheeks. It's a "come hither" makeup for a girl who welcomes the unexpected with open arms.

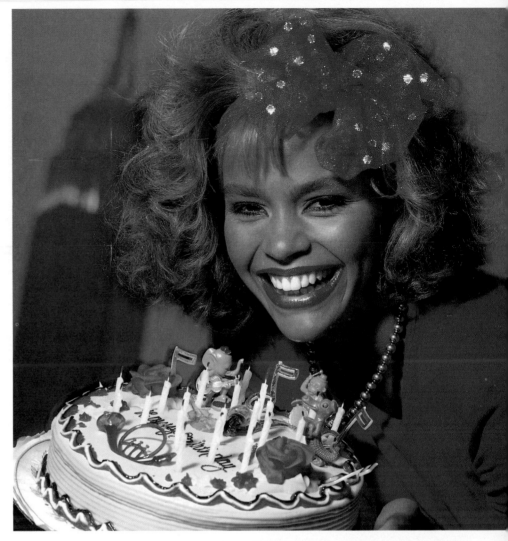

# EVENING

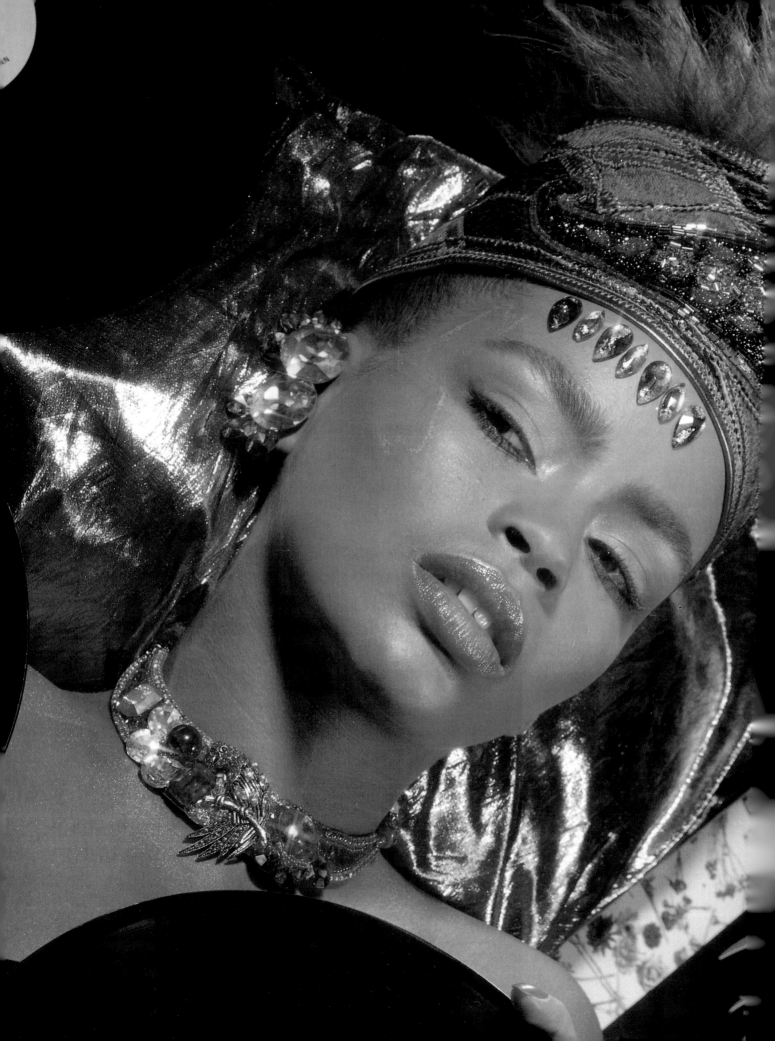

Here Kersti sheds all her inhibitions with a daring special effects makeup. Her motto is "I can do anything"—and she shows it, transforming herself into an exotic queen of the night with a combination of makeup and fashion accessories that spans the colors of the rainbow. There's color everywhere—eyes (gold/mango/lime/pink shadows, coconut shaping pencil, cognac liner, and red mascara); lips (orange pencil, mango powder, gypsy-orange lipstick, gold highlighter dust); and face (orange/mango/golden bronze). And as for special effects: The design on her cheek is drawn first with a lavender pencil, then traced alongside (using the card/airbrush technique and a powder brush) with two colorful lines of shadows, and completed with a gold glitter gel drawn with an eyeliner brush along the line of pencil. The green, yellow, and blue stones that crown Kersti's forehead (applied with tweezers and eyelash adhesive) are fabulous found objects. And with a headdress, a choker, and earrings to match, Kersti is ready for an unforgettable walk on the wild side.

# NIGHTPLAY

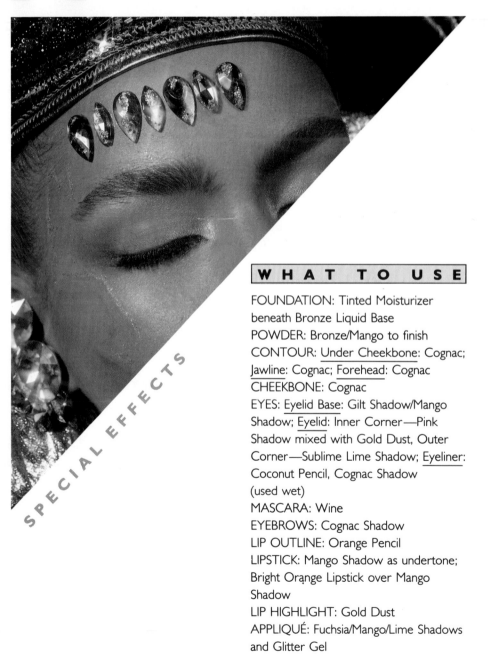

SPECIAL EFFECTS

## WHAT TO USE

FOUNDATION: Tinted Moisturizer beneath Bronze Liquid Base
POWDER: Bronze/Mango to finish
CONTOUR: Under Cheekbone: Cognac; Jawline: Cognac; Forehead: Cognac
CHEEKBONE: Cognac
EYES: Eyelid Base: Gilt Shadow/Mango Shadow; Eyelid: Inner Corner—Pink Shadow mixed with Gold Dust, Outer Corner—Sublime Lime Shadow; Eyeliner: Coconut Pencil, Cognac Shadow (used wet)
MASCARA: Wine
EYEBROWS: Cognac Shadow
LIP OUTLINE: Orange Pencil
LIPSTICK: Mango Shadow as undertone; Bright Orange Lipstick over Mango Shadow
LIP HIGHLIGHT: Gold Dust
APPLIQUÉ: Fuchsia/Mango/Lime Shadows and Glitter Gel

# TINA LITTLEWOOD:

# ALL-AMERICAN BLONDE

Tina is the beautiful girl next door, a healthy California blonde with the knack of looking sophisticated and natural at the same time. She lives near the beach and adores the outdoors, spending a lot of time in and around the water, but she also dreams of being a Hollywood star and consequently revels in glamour as well.

She keeps her makeup light, most of the time preferring a natural look to show off her clear skin and glowing tan. She even accomplishes a more urbane look with relatively little makeup. Breaking the color barrier is her way to keep her makeup minimal while packing it with eye-catching power. So when she wants to feel special (even at the beach), she often does it with a touch of melon, a hint of lavender, a splash of green instead of her basic browns and blues.

Freckles sometimes develop along with Tina's tan. Scrupulous use of a sunscreen can minimize them, but once they're there it's too late. So when the occasion calls for it, Tina wears foundation to tone down the tan and cover the freckles. She also uses makeup to raise and arch her eyebrows—helping her to open up the lids around the outer part of her eyes. And makeup always helps her to explore the possibilities of who she is.

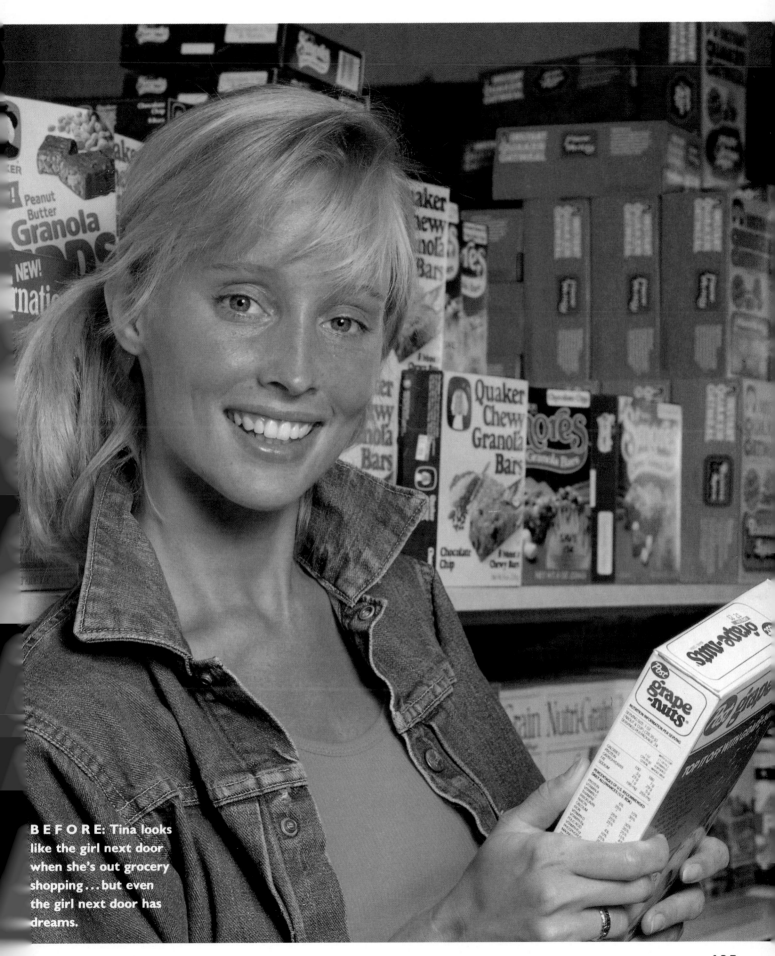

**BEFORE:** Tina looks like the girl next door when she's out grocery shopping...but even the girl next door has dreams.

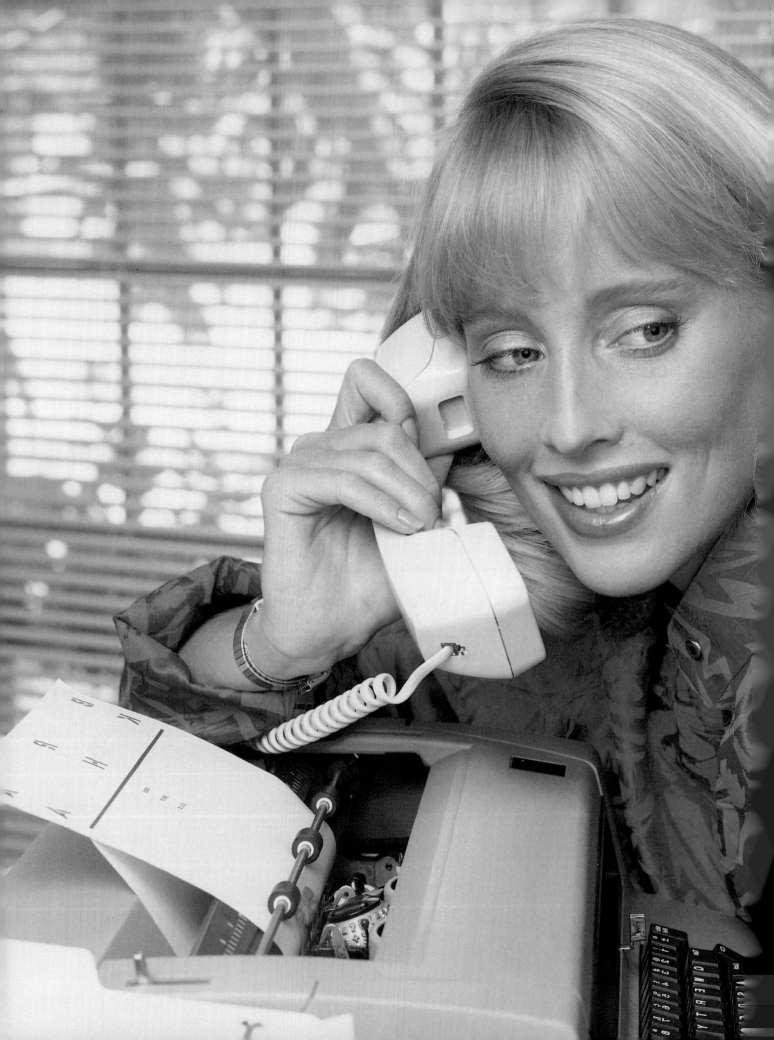

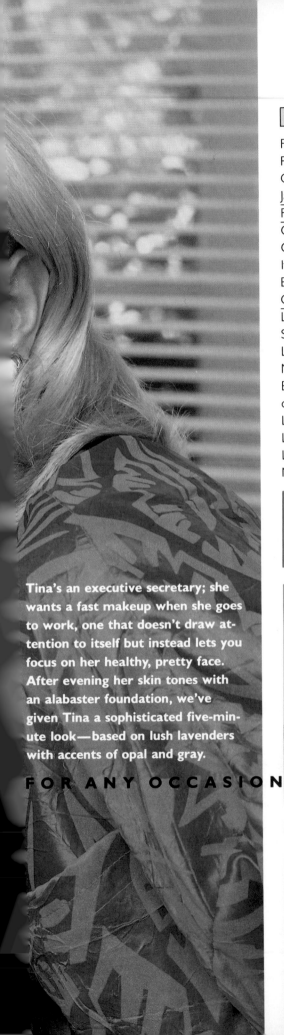

## WHAT TO USE

FOUNDATION: Porcelain Liquid Base
POWDER: Porcelain
CONTOUR: Under Cheekbone: Taupe;
Jawline: Taupe; Nose: Taupe;
Forehead: Taupe
CHEEKBONE: Bride's Pink
CHEEKBONE HIGHLIGHTS:
Ivory Shadow
EYES: Eyelid Base: Ivory Shadow; Eye
Contour: Lavender Shadow; Eyeliner:
Lavender Pencil; Eyelid: Inner Corner—
Snow Shadow, Outer Corner—
Lavender Shadow
MASCARA: Brown
EYEBROWS: Gray Pencil; Brow Set
over it
LIP OUTLINE: Ginger Pencil
LIPSTICK: Opal
LIP GLOSS: Pearl
NAILS: Pale Pink

# DAYTIME

Tina's an executive secretary; she wants a fast makeup when she goes to work, one that doesn't draw attention to itself but instead lets you focus on her healthy, pretty face. After evening her skin tones with an alabaster foundation, we've given Tina a sophisticated five-minute look—based on lush lavenders with accents of opal and gray.

## FOR ANY OCCASION

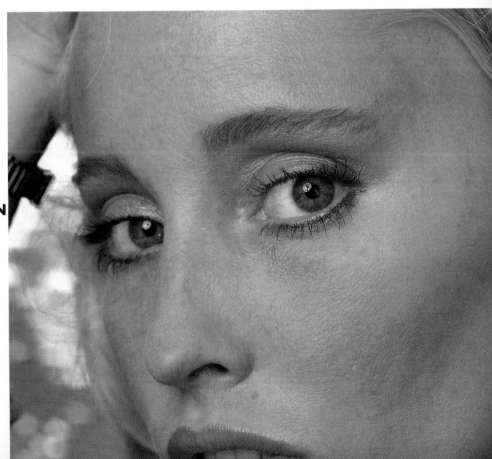

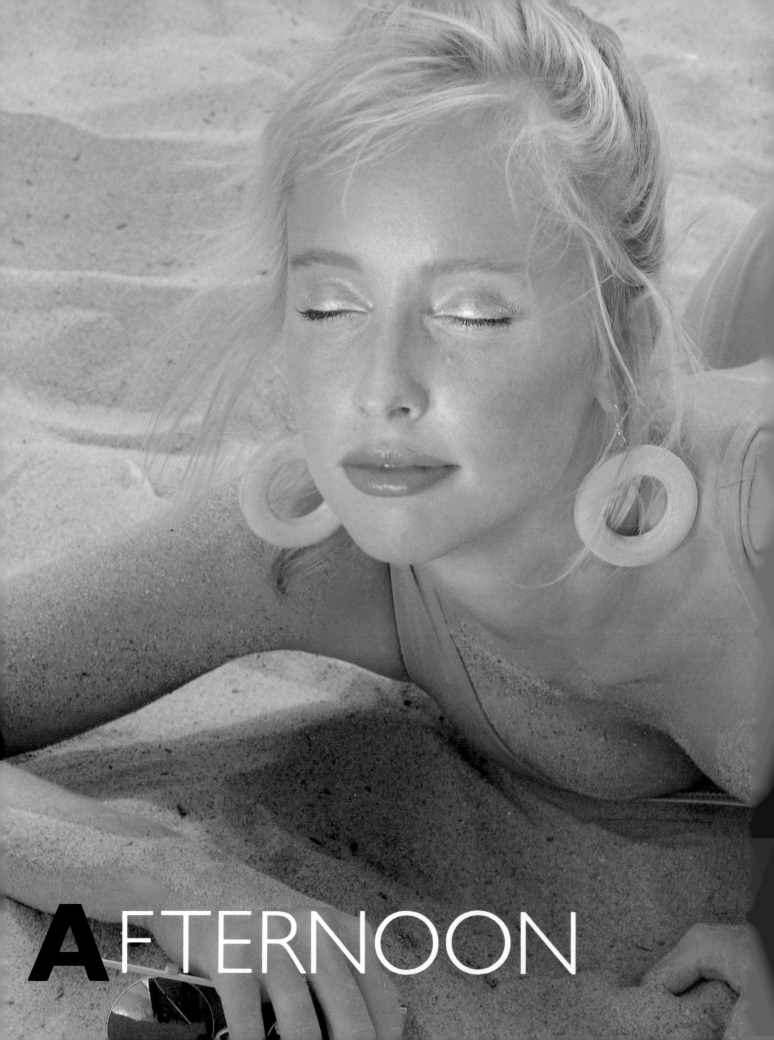

AFTERNOON

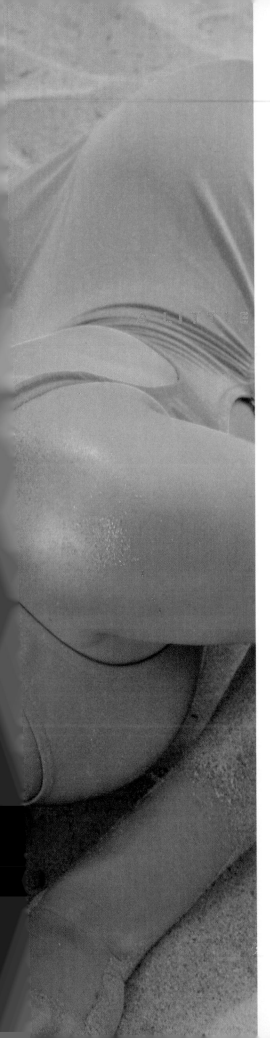

SOPHISTICATION

Who would think that a sunbathing makeup could be so sophisticated? Here's a truly minimal makeup, one that uses a sunscreen on the face and all over the body as a moisturizer/foundation combination (which allows for a healthy tan but not for freckles and burning). What makes it special is color, the peach shades that light up lips and cheeks, and the sparkling green and neon gilt that frames Tina's eyes.

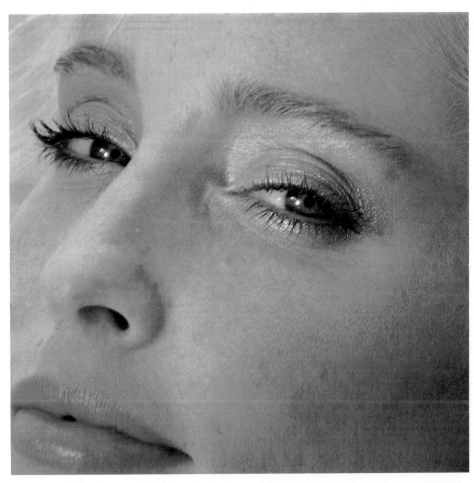

**WHAT TO USE**

FOUNDATION: Sunscreen
CHEEKBONE: Peach
EYES: <u>Eyelid Base:</u> Gilt Cream Shadow;
<u>Eyeliner:</u> Green Highlighter Dust
(applied wet)
MASCARA: Green
EYEBROWS: Light Brown Shadow
LIP GLOSS: Apricot

# NIGHTPLAY

Tina's a guest at a Hollywood party held aboard a producer's yacht. The colors of her makeup are white, black, and red, a dramatic look that evokes the image of yet another American blonde—Marilyn Monroe.

This is a makeup that looks relatively natural but abounds in special effects. Most spectacularly, we changed the shape of Tina's eyebrows, arching them high for a sensuous look. The method of this transformation: Apply a white cream shadow all over the lids as well as over the entire outer half of the eyebrow; then draw in the new shape with a taupe pencil.

We also created a black beauty mark on Tina's cheek, using a black eyebrow pencil. Here's how: First decide where you want your beauty mark to go and lightly mark the spot; then light a match, hold it for no more than half a second under your pencil point (or just long enough to allow your pencil to melt but *not* to drip); then almost immediately touch the point to the spot you marked.

Other effects—eyes: two pairs of strip eyelashes on top and individual lashes on the bottom; black eyeliner around the outer part of eyes for a wider set. Other effects—lips: red outline drawn under the natural line of the lower lip to make lips fuller, more seductive; and a white iridescent highlighter blended in the center of the lips to make them even more sumptuous. Delicious!

## WHAT TO USE

FOUNDATION: Porcelain mixed with White Toner
POWDER: Porcelain
CONTOUR: Under Cheekbone: Taupe; Jawline: Taupe; Nose: Taupe; Forehead: Taupe
CHEEKBONE: Pale Pink Rouge
EYES: Eyelid Base: White Cream Shadow with White Powder Shadow over it; Eyeliner: Black Cake Liner
MASCARA: Black
EYEBROWS: White Cream Shadow over them; Taupe pencil to draw in a new shape
LIP OUTLINE: Red Pencil
LIPSTICK: Hot Red
LIP HIGHLIGHT: White Dust
EYELASHES: Top—Black Strip Lashes; Bottom—Black Individual Lashes
NAILS: Red

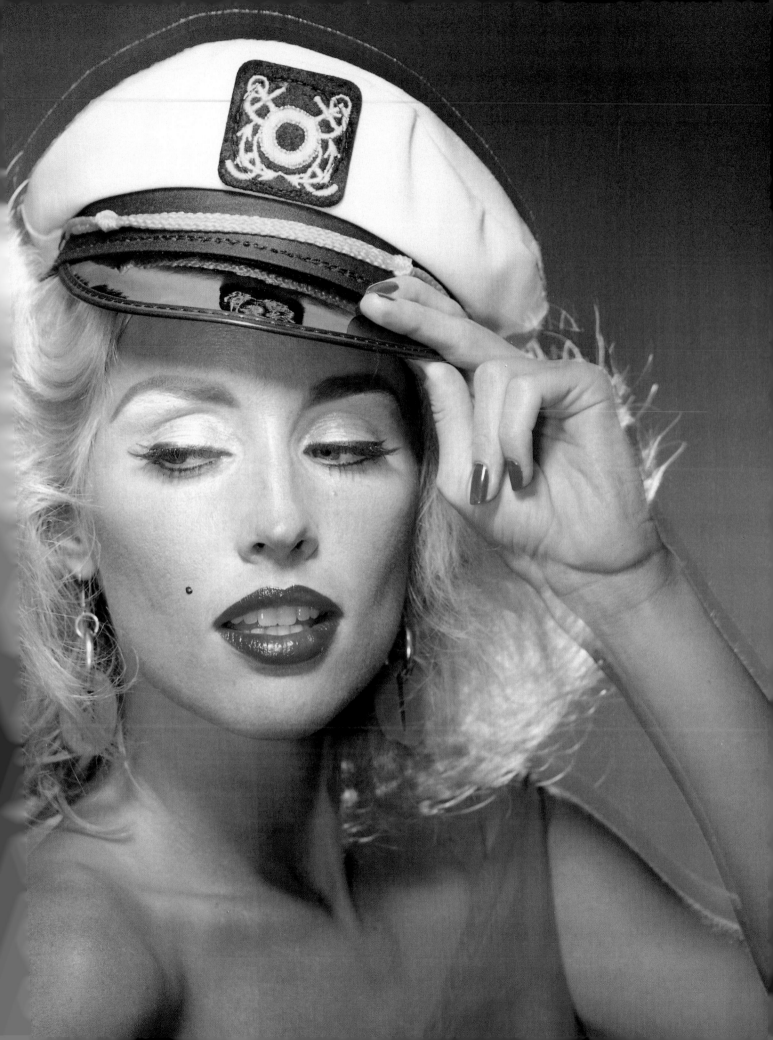

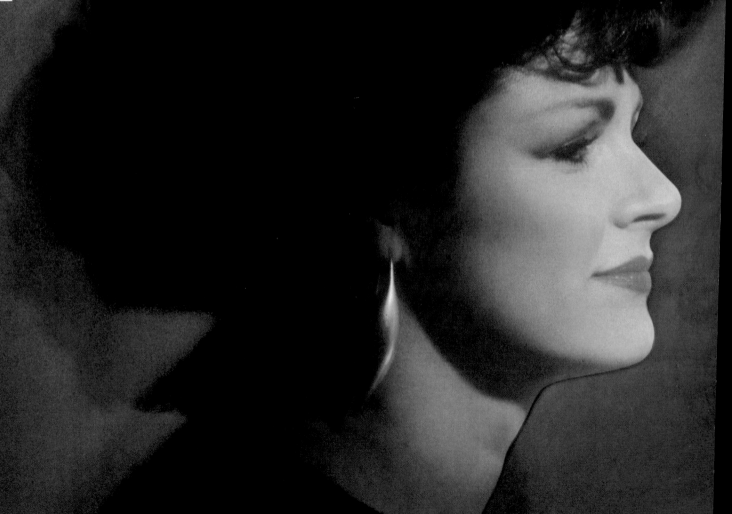

# PART 3

# BEAUTY BASICS

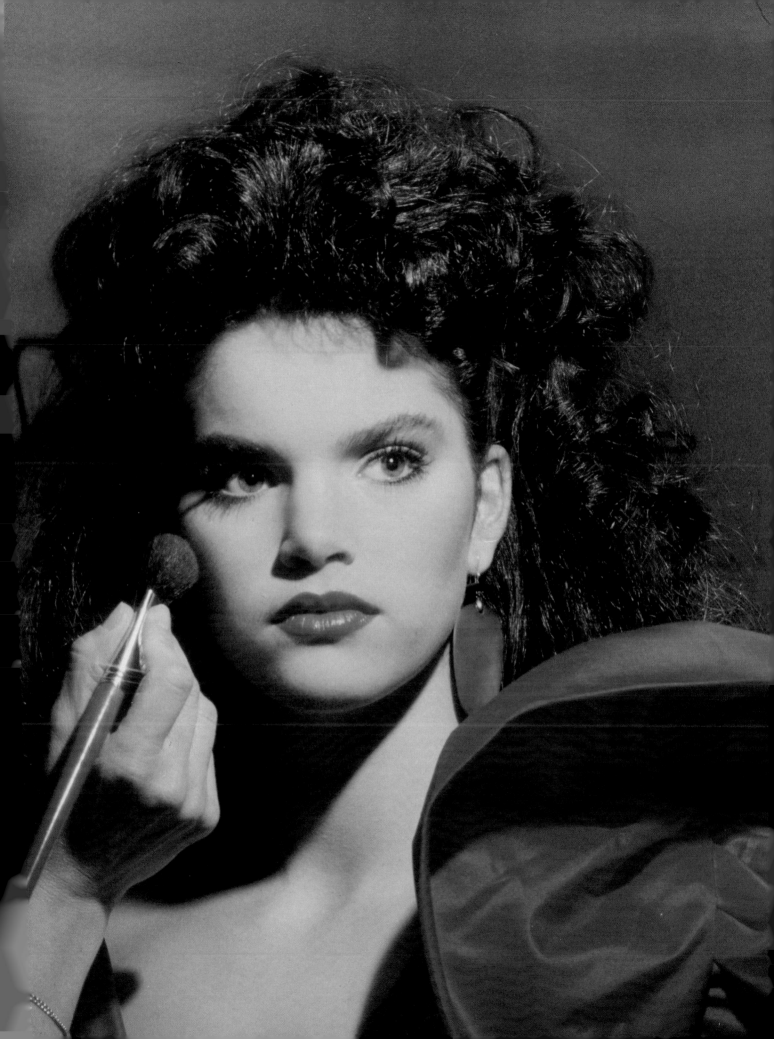

# NATURAL BEAUTY: HEALTHY SKIN

Ask any top model to divulge her most closely guarded beauty secret, and chances are her answer will go *skin deep*. Those gorgeous, glamorous professionals know how contouring can add dimension, how shadows can spark excitement; but when your face is your fortune (and what woman *doesn't* need to put her best face forward every day?) it's what's *underneath* your makeup that counts.

Your complexion is the real foundation of your nat-

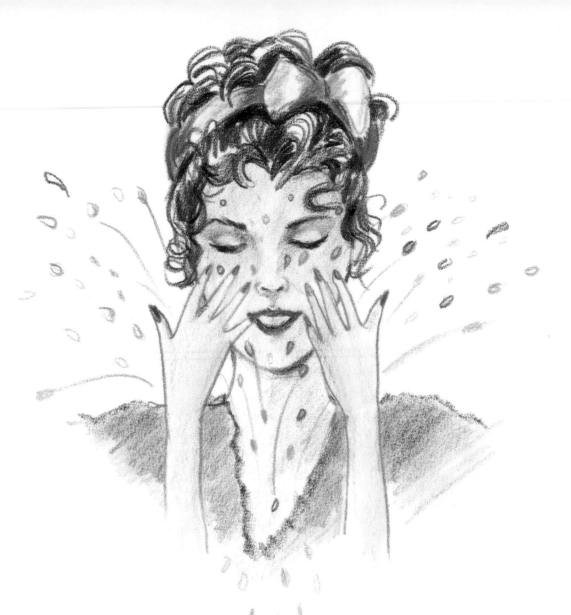

ural beauty, the essence of your uniqueness, and the canvas upon which you create your many looks. Yet, for many women, the clear, clean skin that could be their most important natural asset becomes instead a breeding ground for their biggest beauty problems: blemishes, dryness, blotchiness, and flaking. Yet any skin can be fresh, glowing skin—all it takes is ten minutes of your time each day, and the willingness to take me up on this beauty bargain.

# THE PROPOSITION— AND THE PROMISE

I have a proposition to make—and a promise, too. Take the time to read this chapter. Get to know your skin: how it works, why it looks the way it does, what its enemies are and how to combat them. Find out how your monthly hormonal fluctuations affect your complexion, and learn to compensate for the bad days of your skin cycle. Then commit just ten minutes of your day to a beautiful new you, and I promise that in one week, with a minimum of time, effort, and expense, your skin will feel smoother, look fresher, and be healthier—no matter what your age or skin type. And because the benefits of proper skin care *increase* as time passes, your new regime will not only take years off your face *now*, but will pay big beauty dividends for years to come.

Ready to put a smooth, clear complexion into your immediate future? Then start here with the inside scoop—the story of what's *really* underneath it all.

# THE INSIDE STORY

How deep is "skin deep"? Although you may know your complexion as the surface that you present to the world, your skin is complex enough to protect you from disease and regulate your temperature, sensitive enough to allow you to feel your environment—and deep enough to reach straight to the heart of your genetic beauty bonuses—and complexion woes.

Just a postage-stamp-sized piece of healthy skin contains millions of living, growing cells. These include oil glands, sweat glands, nerve strands, nerve endings, hair follicles, blood vessels, fatty deposits, and collagen fibers—each performing a task crucial to your general well-being.

Healthy skin is in a constant state of transition. The skin you see is just the outermost layer of overlapping, paper-thin cells that push to the surface and are then worn away. Beneath, millions of new skin cells are forming daily to replace those layers that are naturally shed. When your skin is functioning properly, this regeneration process continues twenty-four hours a day, leaving the surface of your skin soft, moist, even-textured—and protected by the delicate acid mantle, nature's own invisible barrier against bacteria.

Beneath the visible layer of skin, which is called the epidermis, lies a much thicker layer known as the dermis. The dermis is the skin's workshop. Here the sebaceous glands produce the natural oils that keep the surface skin moist and protected. Here the skin's blood vessels collect water and nutrients to feed the plump new skin cells and help the skin breathe. And here, too, is the interior scaffolding of the skin—the vast network of collagen and elastin fibers that crisscrosses the dermis, giving the visible skin its texture and firmness.

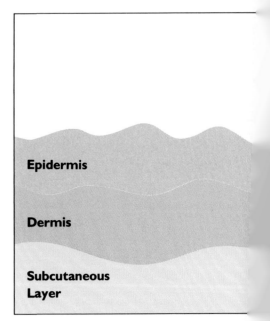

**Epidermis**

**Dermis**

**Subcutaneous Layer**

# THE MANY AGES OF BEAUTY— YOUR SKIN'S LIFE CYCLE

The condition of your complexion, no matter what your age, is determined by a combination of factors, both internal—like heredity, diet, and general health—and external—which includes topical care and tending.

Almost everyone is born with a beautiful complexion—radiant, soft, and healthy. If you're among the lucky few, your skin may continue to glow with just the right amount of natural moisture for the rest of your life. But, by and large, great complexions are made, not born, and as our skin ages, most of us eventually find that we've inherited less-than-perfect complexions from our parents.

Our genetically programmed skin characteristics come to the surface by our early teens when skin is likely to be laden with a considerable amount of moisture.

Natural oils help nurture skin, but when overly abundant, can precipitate acne breakouts. As a result, if you are genetically predisposed to oily skin, you are likely to be plagued with breakouts during your teens—breakouts that may cause permanent scarring unless cared for properly.

Once you've passed your adolescence, your skin stops manufacturing excess oil—blemishes clear and skin becomes more manageable. By their twenties, even women who have endured a serious acne problem in their teens see a marked improvement in their skin, even though it may remain oily. Others may experience excessive oiliness only in the T-zone—across the forehead and along the nose and chin—and dryness in other areas of the face. This is the skin type appropriately known as "mixed" or "combination" skin.

Between twenty-eight and thirty, most complexions change once again. Regardless of skin type, sebaceous glands slow down oil production and skin becomes noticeably drier. Women who suffered throughout their twenties with extremely oily skin now find that their skin is in its best shape ever, while those with mixed skins find that drier areas are now very dry, and the oily areas less shiny than before. This is also when those women with a genetic predisposition toward dry skin (who sailed through their twenties without even a slight eruption) begin dehydrating.

After the age of thirty, the watchword is *preservation*. As skin ages, it becomes drier, less elastic, and, unfortunately, less resistant to lining. While scrupulous skin care can offset and even delay the consequences of aging, the effects of your skin's enemies upon your complexion are *cumulative*—and no regime can undo years of damage once the structure of your skin has begun to deteriorate.

Keep over-thirty skin as moist and supple as possible; when necessary, rejuvenate with collagen treatments. And no matter what your age, plan ahead for perpetually beautiful skin by avoiding your skin's natural adversaries—and begin courting its friends.

# Your Skin's Worst Enemies

**The sun:** The ultimate dehydrator! Expose unprotected skin to the sun's ultraviolet rays and sunburn, and wrinkles,sunspots, premature aging, skin cancer, and permanent damage to the underlying layers could result. **Wind and cold:** Moisture evaporates from skin exposed to harsh weather faster than the body can replace it. The result? Chapping and irritation, premature aging, and permanent lining of the skin.

**Pollution:** Exhaust fumes, street grime, and other pollutants are the bane of urban women—and the cause of blackheads, blemishes, and chronic adult acne.

**Air conditioning and steam heat:** An air conditioner's chilly blasts tighten and dehydrate skin much the way a winter wind does—and steam, though a helpful part of a *brief* skin treatment, drains natural oils and causes skin to sag. Compensate for your environment by drinking plenty of water, moisturizing religiously—and keeping environmental humidity *balanced*.

**Smoking:** An unhealthy habit that sallows skin, slows circulation, and causes wrinkling around lips and eyes.

**Too much coffee, tea, or alcohol:** If you want to play, your skin will pay! Because caffeine and alcohol are diuretics, they force moisture out of your system. Tipple too frequently and your complexion will wrinkle and line—while too much caffeine can cause skin color to yellow.

**Hot water and harsh soaps:** No skin type benefits from overly zealous cleansing! Washing with hot water and the wrong soap scalds skin, undermines the natural acid mantle, and can cause broken capillaries. Even oily complexions can become dehydrated from overuse of hot water and soap, causing oils to collect under taut, dry surface skin. Subject dry skin to this tortuous regime and it will wrinkle and line.

**An inadequate diet:** Why do models munch on fresh "live foods" (crisp, raw vegetables and fruits) rather than overprocessed snacks and red meats? Because overrefined, starchy foods contribute to tired, lifeless skin. Although fried foods, spices, and sugars *don't* cause acne (your mother was wrong!), neither do they supply the nutrients that encourage cell regeneration. And because red meats digest very slowly, frequent meat-eaters have systems that metabolize more slowly. The result? A sluggish turnover of new skin cells, a dull complexion, and poor skin tone.

**Stress:** Sagging skin, discoloration, lines, wrinkles, and blemishes—all are potential consequences of too much pressure and too little relaxation.

**Lack of sleep:** Exhaustion shows up first in the delicate skin around the eyes. After even one sleepless night this thin skin may look creased and puffy or may be marred by dark undereye circles.

**Lack of exercise:** When circulation slows down due to lack of exercise, fewer nutrients feed the skin. Soon, the regeneration process languishes.

**Habitual facial gestures:** Repeated squinting, frowning, pouting, and "talking with your face" exaggerate lines and wrinkles, eventually causing expressions to etch their way permanently into the skin.

**Your own hands:** Every time you rub or pull at your face or cradle your chin, you are spreading dirt and bacteria from your fingers, stretching delicate skin out of shape, and encouraging broken capillaries. Even habitually cradling the telephone on your chin can damage your skin—and lead to blemish flare-ups.

## Your Skin's Best Friends

• Use a protective **sunscreen** (the higher the SPF factor the better!) any time you are directly exposed to the sun to discourage drying, wrinkling, and skin cancer. After your mid-twenties, stay out of the sun as much as possible to keep your complexion wrinkle-free.

• A well-chosen **moisturizer** forms a protective barrier between pollution, the elements, and your skin. Use one formulated for your skin type every day to slow natural moisture loss and, consequently, the aging process.

• When showering, use **tepid water** and a **mild cleansing soap**. Gentle cleansing is just as thorough and less destructive to your skin's natural acid mantle than hot water and harsh soap.

• A **healthy diet** supplies nutrients and moisture to the skin, keeping regenerative powers high. Treat dry skin from the inside out by feasting on foods rich in Vitamin A, like cantaloupe, yogurt, and olive and safflower oils. Vitamin C-rich foods, like citrus fruits, strawberries, and green peppers, rev up collagen production, which keeps skin supple. Wheat germ and whole-grain cereals reduce stress and promote healing. Remember: You *are* what you eat!

• **Drink six to eight glasses of water every day**. Water is nature's perfect moisturizer: Drink it in! You'll speed cell growth, improve circulation, and flush any impurities out of your system—and your skin will look fresher and clearer in just ten days.

• **Take the worry off your face** and your skin will look younger immediately. Become aware of those habitual expressions that can permanently line your skin. And when you catch yourself frowning or furrowing your brow, relax your facial muscles and take a few deep cleansing breaths.

• **Exercise regularly** to revive circulation and speed blood to the surface of your skin. That healthy post-exercise glow is a sign that your heart and lungs are working to regenerate your skin. Besides, exercise helps you sleep better.

• And before you go to sleep, take a moment to relax the muscles of your face—then **sleep** as long as you need to. Remember, models get seven to eight hours of sleep every night.

• Finally, **treat your skin with respect**. Never clean it with harsh solutions or gritty substances, which can burn or scratch the epidermis. Use your *clean* hands to pamper your skin, not abuse it. And to keep your complexion glowing, use only those skin-care preparations specifically formulated for your skin type.

# YOUR SKIN TYPE: TO KNOW IT IS TO LOVE IT

Though your blemish-prone complexion may seem a nuisance, your flaking skin a constant frustration, take heart: *Your* skin, no matter what its problems, has the potential to become *great* skin once you really get to know it, inside and out.

Every skin type has its redeeming qualities—the oily complexion that may now be your burden is likely to remain moist longer, resisting wrinkles as you age. With proper care, dry skin can be enviably poreless and even-textured, with a porcelainlike finish. And even mixed skin can be balanced, so that oily T-zone shine becomes a healthy glow. But to really make the most of your skin's best qualities—and to minimize its other traits—you must first understand your complexion. And that skin-deep understanding begins with an accurate analysis.

Although the size of your pores is a clue to your inherited skin type—clusters of visible pores can mean your skin is oily; tiny, nearly invisible pores denote dry skin—seeing is not always believing, particularly when you scan the surface of your skin with an uneducated eye. Oily, large pore areas in the T-zone have led thousands of women to treat their combination skin with harsh drying agents that dehydrate forehead, nose, and chin while devastating delicate, dry cheeks. And I can't tell you how many times a client has complained to me about the acne that will not respond to over-the-counter medication, only to discover that her skin is actually dry, sensitive, and so irritated that it has been chafed into a perpetual rash.

Using the *wrong* skin-care preparations can be as damaging to your skin as using no skin-care preparations at all! Begin *any* skin-care regime without carefully analyzing your skin type and you run the risk of dehydrating already taut, dry skin, breaking capillaries, and clogging sluggish pores. But take the time to analyze your skin type now and you'll see your complexion for what it really is; then use that information as the basis of a personalized skin-care program that will make your complexion glow! Keep up with the changes in your skin's tone and texture by repeating your analysis every six months and your skin will *always* be at its beautiful best.

## The Blotter Test

This test always works, but to ensure the most accurate results, do it when hormones are most stable, at the end of the third week of your menstrual cycle. All you need is a notepad and pencil for record keeping, and three transparent cigarette rolling papers (or permanent wave papers, the thin tissues hairdressers use to protect the ends of your hair from waving solutions).

Wash or cleanse your face as usual. Because any soap or cleanser is going to be fairly alkaline, wait two hours for the acid mantle to reappear on your skin or your skin will seem less oily than it actually is.

Enumerate one, two, and three on your notepad. Then press paper number one against the center of your forehead and blot the skin slightly. With the second paper, blot the sides of the nose and the center of the chin. Finally, use the remaining piece of paper to blot the cheeks, and place the three papers in front of you to compare their appearance.

The flow of natural oils can differ significantly from forehead to nose to cheeks; blotting with the thin, absorbent paper provides you with tangible (and often surprising) evidence of those differences. A dark stain denotes oiliness. A very oily stain shows that you have overactive sebaceous glands in that area of your face. But if the papers look damp rather than stained, you have a moderate amount of moisture in your skin—your complexion is normal, not oily. No visible stain means that you have little or no surface oil—in other words, dry skin.

Sometimes all three papers present a fairly uniform appearance, either because the skin is generally dry or generally oily. Be sure to check each paper carefully even when they all look pretty much the same: It may be helpful to know that your dry skin is even drier in certain areas or that your oily skin needs more attention in the T-zone area, where excess moisture can be most troublesome. Then jot the results of your analysis into your notebook for a map of your problem areas.

## Oily Skin

When all three of your blotter papers come away with dark stains, and large pores are visible to the naked eye, your skin is generally oily in all three areas of your face.

Because natural oils constantly flow to the surface, oily skin and large pore areas must be kept scrupulously clean to keep that greasy shine from breaking through your makeup—and to keep blemishes at bay. But keep soaps and other cleansing agents away from the delicate skin around your eyes; this fragile area has *no* oil glands and it will dry out before the rest of your skin—adding ten years to your look.

The challenge of oily skin is to *maintain* it without overdrying it. But caring properly for an oily complexion pays beauty dividends that can last a lifetime. Oily skin may be a nuisance when you're twenty, but it's a blessing when you're forty.

## Mixed or Combination Skin

If you find yourself writing "oily, oily, and dry" in your skin notepad, you have a skin type shared by eight out of ten American women between the ages of twenty and thirty—mixed or combination skin.

Most of the time, combination skin means normal cheeks with an oily T-zone, but occasionally mixed skin appears as a band of oily skin across the upper part of the face and a band of normal skin across the cheeks and chin.

Because the difference between dry and oilier areas can be extreme—such as an excessively oily T-zone and very taut, dry cheeks—the key to coping with combination skin is *balancing* or normalizing all the skin types of the face. Buy skin-care products especially formulated for normal, dry, or combination skin and you'll nourish taut, flaky areas; then spot treat oily areas with tonics, masks, and cleansers as needed. And don't forget to use a moisturizer for the dry skin around your eyes.

## Dry Skin

If none of the three papers has picked up even a spot of oil, your skin is dry, but that isn't where your skin analysis should stop! There are two types of dry skin: *oil-dry skin*, a fairly common condition resulting from the improper functioning of the oil glands, and *oil-gland-dry skin*, a more extreme condition symptomized by sensitivity to heat, cold, and environmental irritants, tightly closed, nearly impenetrable pores, and prematurely lined skin.

Oil-dry skin is really moisture-dry, resulting from a combination of inactive sebaceous glands and weathering by the elements. It generally becomes noticeable in one's late teens or early twenties. Because oil-dry skin needs both internal and external moisturizing, be sure to drink plenty of water each day—then seal in the benefits of your inside/outside skin program by using a moisturizer day and night. Flakiness will disappear—and you will be left with a classic porcelain complexion, clear, fresh, and even-textured.

If no moisture at all comes off on your test papers, if tiny, red broken capillaries are visible beneath the surface of the skin, and if your skin feels uncomfortably (and *consistently*) dry and taut, chances are you have dry and sensitive or oil-gland-dry skin. Because this skin type is nearly impenetrable by creams, as a result of pore tightness, dry and sensitive skin can become *problem* skin. Natural oils cannot flow through the pores to the skin's surface, and moisturizers cannot penetrate to relieve the skin's tightness. Furthermore, heavy emollients, often sought out by women with oil-gland-dry skin, can make the skin perspire, leading to clogged pores.

Because this skin type is hypersensitive, creams used to relieve the tautness can irritate the skin, as can extreme changes in temperature. Never splash hot or cold water on oil-gland-dry skin or sit in a sauna or steam room: Broken capillaries can result and your skin can remain red for hours. Instead, wash gently in tepid water with an extremely mild, hypoallergenic cleanser. And drink as much water as you can—at least eight glasses a day—to counteract tautness and allow natural oils to flow to the skin's surface.

## Acne/Problem Skin

If your blotting papers come away heavily stained with oil, if blemishes of one kind or another are almost always visible on the surface of your skin, you have unusually oily or acne/problem skin.

While young skin with an overabundance of natural oils is most prone to breakouts, acne/problem skin can endure well into adulthood, particularly when environmental problems such as pollution or stress aggravate the condition. But blemishes can be deceiving—rashes can be mistaken for acne when they have nothing to do with your skin's excessive oiliness. If you break out in small, red blotches, cautiously and gently investigate the skin around the rash with clean fingers. If it feels dry and scaly, consult a dermatologist.

Acne/problem skin requires a special cleansing regimen to keep it free of oil without irritating or overdrying it. Oily skin is not "tough" skin—your blemishes are evidence of your skin's sensitivity, so be careful not to scour it. Overly zealous cleansing can aggravate the condition you are trying to quell.

## Dehydrated Skin

A tight, dry feeling does not necessarily mean that you have dry skin. If you're in your twenties and had oily skin in your teens but now find that the top layer of skin is becoming dry and chapped, chances are that environmental factors have taken their toll on your complexion. Surface skin that has been dried out by heat, sun, saltwater, harsh chemicals, or the wrong skin-care products is dehydrated skin, not dry skin. Begin moisturizing regularly with a water-based product formulated for normal complexions, and natural oils will begin to make their way to the surface—and you will be better equipped to determine your skin's true type and condition.

## Dry on Top, Oily Underneath

**T**ry to combat oily skin with harsh drying agents and soaps, and this condition is sure to result. Over-the-counter acne preparations can dehydrate surface skin to the point of peeling, but they cannot reach sebaceous deposits underneath. If the visible layer of your oily skin is taut and dry but you can feel bumps (even cysts) forming underneath, your skin-care preparations are contributing to your complexion woes. Stop overdrying your skin by switching to a milder cleanser, then encourage natural oils and sebaceous deposits to flow to the surface of your skin by drinking six glasses of water every day and using a greaseless moisturizer formulated for your skin type. Meanwhile, exfoliate with a facial scrub twice a week to speed skin regeneration, and follow with a mild mask to soothe and heal blemishes.

Regular, gentle cleansing will clean away bacteria and prevent blackheads from forming, especially if you concentrate your efforts on any areas of large pores. Large-pore areas can be further controlled by gently sloughing with a mild skin scrub, then concealed with water-based makeup. But before applying foundation, run an ice cube over your skin to close the pores and leave your skin with a more velvety texture.

## The Final Test: The Elasticity Factor

It is a fact of life: As the complexion ages, the collagen fibers that give skin its elasticity begin to break down. Left unchecked, the deterioration of the skin's "scaffolding" can undermine skin tone and result in a softer, less well-defined jawline. Yet determining the elasticity of your skin literally takes an instant—and working to preserve the substructure that keeps your complexion vital takes only ten minutes each day as part of comprehensive skin-care regime.

To determine elasticity, pinch the jawline in several places. If skin snaps back almost immediately, the elastin and collagen fibers under the surface are still keeping the skin youthful. If skin seems sluggish, switch to collagen-rich skin care products to compensate for the breakdown of your natural fibers (see page 185). Then, to prevent further deterioration, drink plenty of water and *stay out of the sun*. Your tan will last only a short time, but the effects of ultraviolet rays—including damage done to collagen tissues—are permanent.

# SUPER SKIN IN ONE WEEK

Now that you've made a commitment to a beautiful new you, analyzed your skin type, and determined the condition of your complexion, it's time to take the final step and begin the skin-care program that will take your complexion from drab to dynamic in just one week—in less time each day than it took you to learn the inside story of your skin!

By now, most of you have probably tried just about everything to make the most of your complexion—and the least of your skin problems. You've sampled an array of products from cleansers to peels to drying agents that look better in the ads than they do on your face; you've

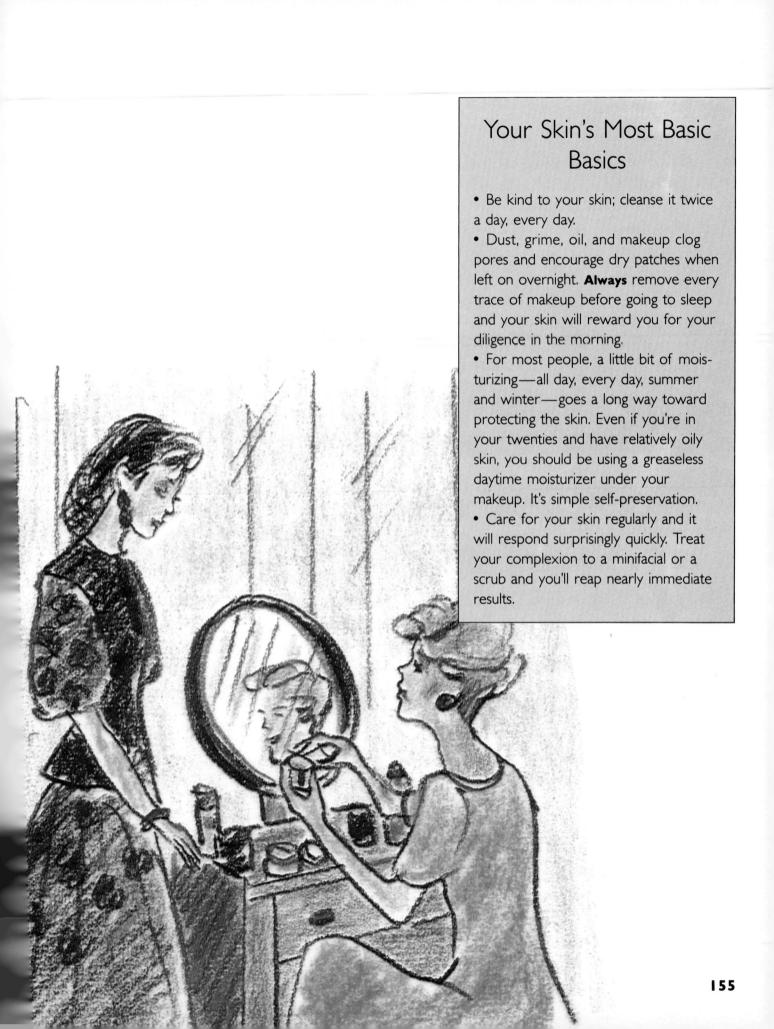

## Your Skin's Most Basic Basics

• Be kind to your skin; cleanse it twice a day, every day.

• Dust, grime, oil, and makeup clog pores and encourage dry patches when left on overnight. **Always** remove every trace of makeup before going to sleep and your skin will reward you for your diligence in the morning.

• For most people, a little bit of moisturizing—all day, every day, summer and winter—goes a long way toward protecting the skin. Even if you're in your twenties and have relatively oily skin, you should be using a greaseless daytime moisturizer under your makeup. It's simple self-preservation.

• Care for your skin regularly and it will respond surprisingly quickly. Treat your complexion to a minifacial or a scrub and you'll reap nearly immediate results.

spent time and money choosing creams that compounded your beauty woes rather than solved them; and you've taken the advice of everyone, from your best friend to the editor of your favorite magazine. Confusing? Of course. Helpful? Not if you're *still* searching the cosmetic counters of your local department store for the answers to your skin-care questions. Isn't it time you confronted the best authority on your complexion face-to-face?

# YOUR SKIN-TYPE ANALYSIS: THE FINAL WORD

If your blotter test revealed that your oily skin is surface-dehydrated yet still troubled by blemishes, if your dry, flaky patches are still craving moisture, the costly preparations that are cluttering up your medicine cabinet have *not* paid off in beauty benefits. Nor are they likely to until you understand this basic tenet of skin care: *Less is more.*

# KEEP IT SIMPLE

How simple can a successful skin-care regime be? Simple enough to meet your needs—to save you both time and money—and well-targeted enough to meet the needs of your skin. Good skin doesn't require limitless time or a dressing table full of bottles and jars. With just a few carefully chosen products and a few minutes of your time each day your skin will regain its glow, as long as you get down to basics.

# THE SKIN-CARE STARTER KIT

Three (yes, just three!) products are the backbone of a daily skin-care program:

The first is a hardworking yet gentle **cleansing lotion**. I recommend a lotion rather than a cream, since creams are too heavily formulated for most skin types and tend to clog the pores.

The second is a **tonic** especially formulated for your skin type. If you have oily skin, use an astringent tonic with as much as 10 percent alcohol. If you have dry skin, use a tonic containing less than 1 percent alcohol. A good tonic not only removes the residue of cleanser, perspiration, and oil, but helps restore the skin's acid mantle as well.

The third is a deep-penetrating **moisture lotion**. All skin types, even oily complexions, need moisturizer—not only to help normalize the skin but to add a protective barrier against the elements and environmental pollution. If your skin is normal to dry,

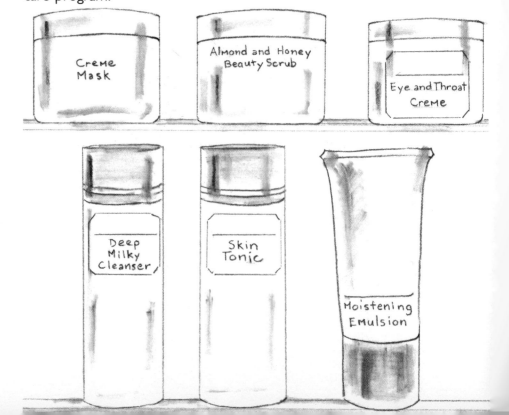

Creme Mask

Almond and Honey Beauty Scrub

Eye and Throat Creme

Deep Milky Cleanser

Skin Tonic

Moistening Emulsion

you must use a moisturizer during the day every day to seal in the natural oils wind and weather can steal. If your skin is oily, a greaseless or water-based moisturizer will guard against surface dehydration in sun or cold weather.

## Other Beauty Boosters

If you're over twenty-five or can see the first signs of dry or lined skin in the delicate areas around your eyes, you will also need a thick penetrating cream to nourish this fragile skin. Add this to your skin-care starter kit to stop laugh lines from etching permanently into your skin.

Although sunscreen technically is not a skin-care product, it is an invaluable addition to your starter kit. Keep it on hand to help you "save face" in sunny weather. And don't forget to treat your arms, neck, and other exposed areas to a healthy coat of sunscreen. You'll stop wrinkles before they start—and prevent freckles and other skin discolorations, as well.

## Occasional Treats

There are two other products you will want to use twice a week to rev up your skin's regeneration process: a skin scrub (or exfoliant) to slough off dead skin cells, and a mask, to revitalize and tone. The type of mask you choose will depend on your skin type.

# BUY WHAT'S RIGHT FOR YOU

I do recommend emollient night creams and day creams—but not for everyone. Young skin needs to breathe at night and doesn't require heavy moisturizing during the day. Too often, a skin-care product formulated for older skin is advertised as if it were for younger women. Don't be bullied into thinking you have to spend a fortune on your skin when your collagen fibers are still vital. Save the super-rich emollients for when your skin needs added protection, or you will risk overloading your skin, clogging your pores and subjecting yourself to allergic rashes.

The wrong products can be particularly dangerous for dry and sensitive skins. Abrasive scrubs can scratch or cause broken capillaries:

harsh, drying, or allergenic ingredients can result in scaly red rashes. Treat your sensitive skin with sensitivity: Use a gentle touch when smoothing on creams and lotions, and never massage your face. And be sure to treat your hypersensitive skin to hypoallergenic skin-care products to avoid eruptions.

Unless you have oily or acne/problem skin, avoid products that contain alcohol, which is too drying for most skins. Always read the label before purchasing any skin-care product.

And never judge a product by its scent. Products that contain chemically produced perfumes and additives can spark allergic reactions even in those with normally nonsensitive skins. If a severe rash or red, flaky patches suddenly appear on your skin, stop using the product immediately—then wash your face with clear water several times a day for at least two days, and drink plenty of water to flush out impurities. To avoid the problem completely, opt for products that are biologically based and scented with an organic perfume (distilled from flowers and herbs) or contain no added scent at all. Inevitably, the products that work best on skin are those that contain the fewest chemicals.

Women often buy their skin-care products hummingbird-style: a cleanser here, a tonic there, and a "moisturizing breakthrough" somewhere else. Mixing products from different skin-care lines is only asking for trouble; ingredients may conflict *violently*. Better to change everything every six months than to risk allergic reactions from the mix of perfumes and other ingredients.

Skin needs time to get used to something new. Give any new product a few days to work before judging it; you may still have traces of a previous product on your skin. Cross-reactions—like mild blemishes or tiny dry patches—often disappear once the skin has fully absorbed a new cream or lotion.

And finally, when choosing products for your ten-minute regimen, remember that a product's shelf life is generally less than six months. The ingredients in creams and lotions can break down—and applying "old" products to your new clear, fresh complexion can be devastating. Don't buy large sizes unless you use the product regularly, and never leave emollient creams in the bathroom where steam can damage them. Instead, keep a small amount on hand and store the rest in a cool, dry place.

# THE IL-MAKIAGE FIVE-MINUTE MORNING SKIN-CARE PROGRAM

Your body cleans itself out while you sleep. Part of the residue of this natural cleansing process is a film of dead cells, salt, and oil left on the surface of your skin. The basic morning program helps you prepare your skin for the day ahead by cleaning away accumulations of excess moisture and worn skin cells, rousing circulation, and revving your complexion to a healthy glow. It's suitable for all skin types.

You will need only three products: a mild soap or milky cleanser, a tonic or astringent formulated for your skin type, and a moisturizer.

(Those with acne/problem skin will need an anti-acne clarifying lotion instead of a moisturizer; those with very dry or dry and sensitive skin will require an emollient day cream as well as a moisturizer.)

## Before You Begin...

Before you even step into the shower, drink a large glass of water with a little lemon juice in it. This early-morning refresher will replenish the fluids you lost while you slept and break up the accumulation of oil and fats in the body. Remember, external skin-care products work hardest only

## About Soap and Water

Many women don't use cleanser, opting for soap and water instead. Most even use the same harsh soaps on their faces that they use on their bodies, leading to prematurely dry skin and possible allergic reactions to chemical additives.

The *only* soaps suitable for cleaning facial skin are complexion bars formulated from biological ingredients or nonfoaming "soapless" soaps. Liquid soaps, which do not contain solidifiers, are also much less hard on the skin.

If you have oily or combination skin, try alternating cleansing milk and soapless soap to combat excessive oiliness and refresh your skin—but never cleanse with detergent-based soaps. Surface dehydration can trap oil beneath the skin, causing blemishes, whiteheads, and even cysts.

Dry skin? Cleanse only with a milky lotion. But don't forget your moisturizer.

when you have enough internal moisture to keep them working.

## First Step: Cleansing

If you have oily, mixed, or normal-to-dry skin, wash your face with a mild complexion bar or milky cleanser and lukewarm water; if your skin is dry, dispense with soap altogether (it will only dehydrate your face further) and cleanse with a milky dry-skin formula and clear water. If you have very dry or dry and sensitive skin, you will require a cleansing lotion.

Pat—never rub—the face dry with a towel; the thin film of moisture left behind will help hydrate your skin.

## Second Step: Toning

Tonics or astringents penetrate pores and bring the skin's naturally protective acid mantle back to the surface. They also close pores, increasing the protection against dust and dirt—and leaving your complexion looking smoother.

Women with combination skin are often confused about what kind of tonic they should use. If your mixed skin is predominantly oily, use an astringent with 10 percent alcohol. If the area outside your T-zone is very dry and sensitive, use a tonic with a minimum of alcohol.

Very oily skin? Carry a small bottle of astringent in your purse. During lunch or a mid-afternoon break, refresh your T-zone with astringent to reduce break-through shine.

### Using Your Tonic

Thoroughly moisten a dry piece of cotton with tonic. Run the cotton over your neck in swift upward motions. Discard the cotton.

Use a second piece of cotton to apply the tonic to your face, beginning and ending at the jaw-line. Check the cotton periodically to see how soiled it is; discard when necessary.

Finally, moisten a third piece of cotton with tonic and go over the face again to remove any remaining traces of soil and cleanser. Then, check cotton; when it comes away snowy-white, your face is scrupulously clean.

Work carefully around the eyes; tonic, no matter what its formulation, is too drying to be used within the area of the eye-bones where skin is most fragile.

## Third Step: Moisturizing

A daytime moisturizer is one of your skin's greatest allies. It locks in natural moisture and protects your face from the elements and pollution.

Daytime moisturizers range from liquid emollients to heavy day creams. If your skin is oily, combination, or normal-to-dry, choose a liquid or lotion formulated for your skin type. Women with very dry or dry and sensitive skins need more protection and should opt for the more penetrating day creams.

### Using a Moisturizer: The One-Minute Massage

Combine your moisturizing regime with a light massage and you'll tone the muscles of your face and put circulation in high gear while you protect your skin. Follow the instructions for using a moisturizer in "The Makeup Lesson" section of this book (page 19). Your skin will love you for it!

Finis! In just five minutes, skin is clean but not dry, toned but not taut. And whether you finish with the *il-Makiage* Five-Minute Makeup or use the time you've saved on skin care to smooth on more dramatic colors to brighten your day, your complexion will glow until you're ready to take it all off.

# THE IL-MAKIAGE FIVE-MINUTE EVENING SKIN-CARE PROGRAM

No regime is more important than this super-cleansing program when day is done. By evening, your skin has absorbed makeup and accumulated dust and dirt all day. Take these enemies to bed with you and they penetrate pores even further, causing blemishes and dry, scaly patches that may be difficult to treat.

This basic evening program shows you how to deep-clean your skin and protect sensitive areas from drying out overnight when your metabolism slows. It's suitable for oily, mixed, and normal-to-dry skin types.

You will need four products: a milky cleanser and a tonic, both formulated for your skin type; an eye and throat cream; and a good, allergen-free eye-makeup remover.

Those with acne/problem skin should use an acne-clarifying lotion instead of a tonic.

Those with dry and sensitive skin will need a nighttime moisturizer, as well.

## Tips for Making the Most of Your Skin-Care Regime

• Begin by putting a sufficient quantity of cream, lotion, or scrub to do the job into the palm or onto the back of your hand. And always use a spoon to dip into jars. Fingers spread germs that can cause blackheads and acne. Keep them out of your cosmetics and you'll keep bacteria away from your face.

• I prefer large cotton pads to cotton balls for cleansing and applying tonic; their generous size makes them easier to work with, and since they're designed for use with cosmetics, they're much kinder to the epidermis. *Never* use tissues to apply or remove makeup: Because facial tissues are made from wood fiber, they can scratch and irritate the skin.

• Very soft natural sponges or facial sponges (not to be confused with makeup sponges!) are excellent for cleaning away every last trace of cleanser, but they must be kept scrupulously clean. Wash them immediately after use, and sterilize them **at least** once a week in rubbing alcohol. And don't be afraid to throw them away once they become worn looking.

## First Step: Cleansing

Soap and water won't do the job adequately: Only cleansers are especially formulated to dissolve oil and dirt and remove makeup without drying. Any woman who uses makeup, no matter how light, should opt for a good cleansing lotion to deep-clean her skin at night.

Use a milky cleansing lotion rather than cold cream. Cold creams are wonderful for dissolving makeup but aren't effective dirt removers. In addition, the oily residue left by many cold creams can contribute to acne flare-ups.

If you must use soap at night, choose a complexion bar or soapless soap to avoid drying your skin—and use it only after makeup has been removed with cleanser. Not even the best complexion bar can dissolve makeup.

And finally, always use a cleanser in conjunction with a tonic. Cleansers are alkaline and do leave a film on the skin, which can disturb the skin's acid mantle; tonics restore the skin's natural acidity after cleansing, leaving skin toned and protected.

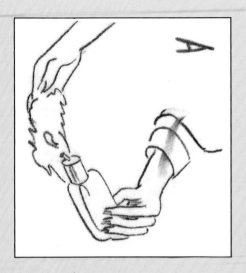

**1.** Begin your thorough cleansing by gently removing eye makeup. Moisten a piece of cotton with hypoallergenic eye-makeup remover.

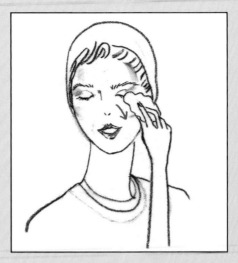

**2.** To remove mascara, close your eye and work the cotton down the lashes.

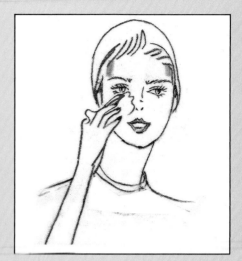

**3.** Clean away residue by working the cotton gently toward the inner corner of the eye. Do not pull!

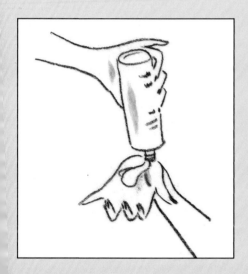

**4.** Wash and dry your hands. Then squeeze a small amount of milky cleanser into the palm of one hand.

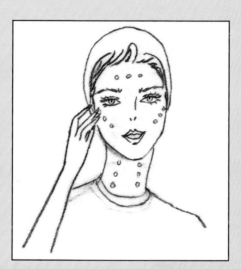

**5.** For an even application, pat three dots of cleanser onto each area of your face: along each cheekbone, across the forehead, and on each side of the neck.

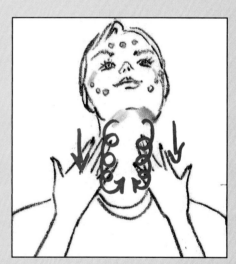

**6.** Using the middle fingers of each hand, blend the cleanser into your neck using sweeping upward motions.

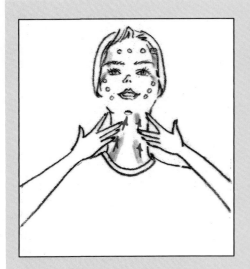

**7.** Further blend into neck using small, circular, downward motions.

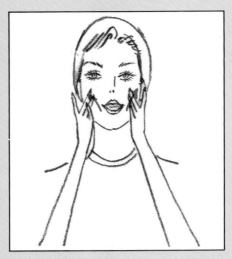

**8.** Blend cleanser into cheeks and around nose. Work with your skin, not against it, by moving fingers in an upward and outward motion.

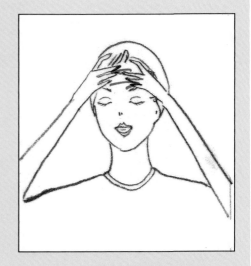

**9.** Blend into forehead by moving fingers back and forth.

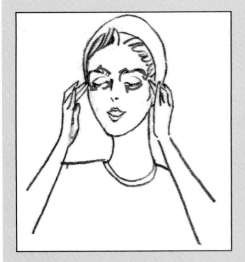

**10.** Use fingertips to gently work cleanser into the skin around the eyes. Work down and in from the outer corner of each eye, then up and out from the inner corner, ending with fingers resting on pressure points just outside the eyebones.

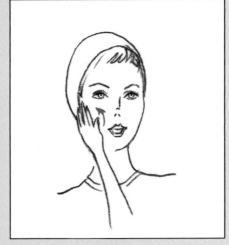

**11.** Blend upward along the outside of your cheeks near your jawline.

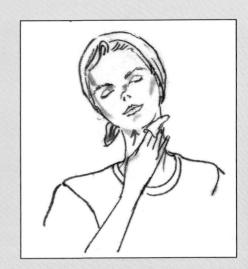

**12.** Dampen a large piece of cotton or a cotton pad. Remove cleanser from neck by working in an upward motion from the base of the neck to the jawline.

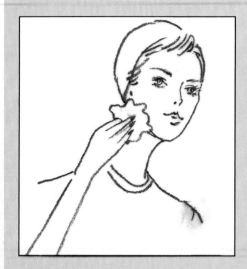

**13.** Remove cleanser from up and under jawline all the way to the tip of the ear.

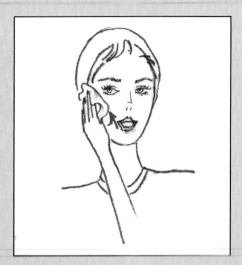

**14.** If you wish, you can also use a facial sponge to remove cleanser.

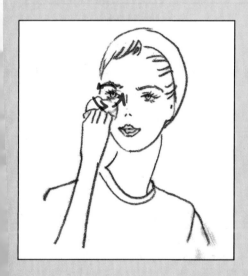

**15.** Remove cleanser from the eye area employing the same circular motion with which you applied it. Be careful to keep the cleanser away from the eyes themselves.

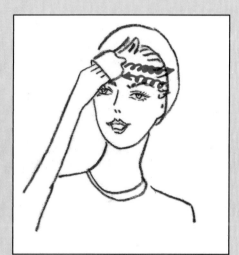

**16.** Remove from forehead by moving cotton back and forth in small circular motions. Complete removing from forehead by using long, upward strokes. Then repeat steps 12 through 16 using a fresh piece of cotton. All the cleanser is removed when your cotton pad stops picking up a gray residue.

## Second Step: Toning

Apply a tonic to help stimulate the pores and to restore the skin's acidity, which the cleansing took away. Go over skin with tonic, discarding soiled cotton, until cotton comes away snowy-white.

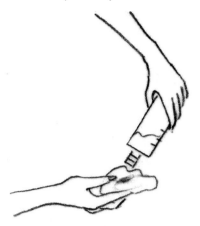

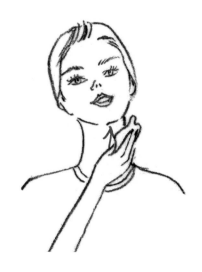

## The Eyes Have It

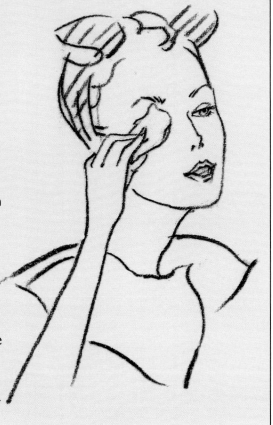

**W**hat do the eyes have? A special glow—and a special makeup-removal problem. The eyes are delicate organs subject to injury and irritation, and they are surrounded by the most fragile skin on your face.

**Never** go to sleep without removing every last trace of mascara and eye shadow. Puffy, irritated lids can result—and fibers from mascara can fall into the eye itself, scratching the cornea.

And **never** try to remove eye makeup with soap and water. Since only specially formulated removers and some natural oils can dissolve mascara and heavy liners, washing with soap will only dry delicate undereye skin *without* cleaning away makeup.

Stroke eye-makeup remover onto lashes and lids with a very light hand, working gently downward to minimize stretching and pulling on fragile skin. And choose a hypoallergenic product to reduce the possibility of inflammation. If skin is oily, look for the new water-based eye-makeup removers; they can be used on even the most moisture-laden skins without rinsing. And if even the mildest commercial preparations irritate your eyes, opt for pure olive oil instead. It penetrates and dissolves even waterproof mascara, leaving the fragile eye area moist, even after rinsing.

## Third Step: Eye and Throat Cream

A deep-penetrating eye cream is one of the best beauty investments you can make. Lines tend to form around the eyes years before they appear elsewhere. Because the paper-thin skin around the eye is easily damaged and almost devoid of moisture-giving sebaceous glands, this area will crease even if you have oily skin.

Dark circles, on the other hand, are the result of pigmentation, iron deficiency, or both. Eye creams soften and protect fragile skin but cannot make dark under-eye circles disappear. Check your iron intake and use a concealer.

Occasionally little white spots appear over the eyelids or under the eye. Consider changing your product; the one you're using may be adding oil but not moisture to the thirsty skin around the eyes.

If you're in your twenties and still have fairly oily skin, you won't need an eye and throat cream every night. Use it on alternate nights or on a daily basis only when the weather is cold.

## Using Eye and Throat Cream

Moisten the back of one hand with a dab of eye cream. (A little of this rich product goes a long way.) Gently apply three dots of cream in a semicircle below each eye, three dots on top of the lip,

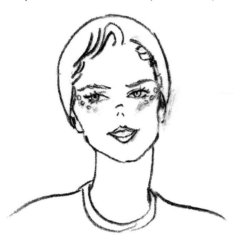

and three dots on each side of the neck.

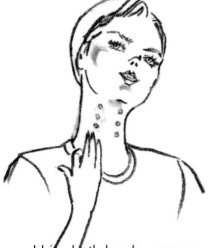

Using both hands, massage the neck with firm, downward sweeping motions. Then use the two middle fingers of each hand to work up the neck in smaller circular motions.

Tap (do not rub!) your two fingers very lightly around eyes and over lids. Work in an outward direction over the eyes and in an inward direction between the eyes so that you don't stretch the skin.

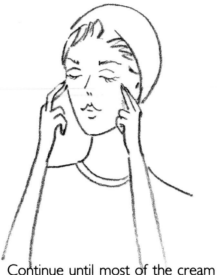

Continue until most of the cream has been absorbed by the skin.

Tap your fingers very lightly along the fragile lip line until the cream has been absorbed.

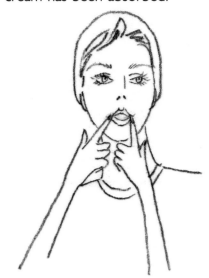

Then use the leftover cream to soothe the backs of your hands, which are often cracked and dry.

If you notice puffiness or a slight irritation around the eyes after using eye and throat cream, the product is too rich for you to leave on overnight. Instead, give the cream ten minutes to penetrate the skin, then blot up the excess. (If irritation still occurs, rinse after blotting, but try to leave as much of the cream as possible.)

Subzero temperatures? Put on eyecream *sparingly* before you go outdoors. Then apply your foundation and powder over it.

## Eye Cream, the All-Around Emollient

**M**assage this rich moisturizer into elbows, knees, and ankles to smooth away rough skin. Rub into the back of the neck to soften that often forgotten area.

Or massage into the skin just above the breasts for silky décolletage.

## Optional Step: Nighttime Moisturizer

Young normal-to-dry, mixed, or oily skin should be allowed to breathe at night, but once you're past thirty, your skin will need an occasional nighttime moisturizing treatment even if it is still fairly oily. Use a nighttime moisturizer formulated for your skin type when cold winds blow or when skin feels taut.

Oily complexions thrive when their nighttime skin treatment contains azulin—a soothing normalizer. But very dry or dry and sensitive skin needs a nourishing night cream every night. Choose a penetrating cream that is enriched with Vitamin E to smooth away dry patches and enhance skin elasticity; blend it in using the technique on page 19. You may even consider taking Vitamin E orally to fight wrinkles from the inside out. (Ask your doctor to recommend the right dosage.)

# **A**CNE: A SPECIAL PROBLEM— AND A SPECIAL REGIME

Most commonly, women with acne problems have young, oily skin. But acne is tenacious, and there are dozens of reasons why you can get it long after your twentieth birthday has passed. The most common time for a breakout is when hormonal levels are unusually elevated just before your period. (See the acne problem skin section of "Your Skin Cycle," page 183, for help during this critical week.) But the use of overly rich skin-care products may also cause eruptions, as can living or working in a polluted environment, high humidity, or emotional upset. In fact, because stress triggers a release of hormones into the bloodstream which closely resembles those that occur in abundance during adolescence, anxiety is probably the single greatest cause of postadolescent acne. Any time your skin can't handle the resulting overabundance of oil you're likely to see an unexpected crop of blemishes.

## A Program for Acne/Problem Skin

When I started working in skin care fourteen years ago, nobody bothered with regimes for blemish-prone skin. They simply covered inconvenient pimples with makeup.

Unfortunately, the pancake makeup most people used as a coverup was a terrible skin irritant—and women found out the hard way that the same makeup that saved them from the embarrassment of blemished skin also spread the problem from one side of the face to the other.

The first cornerstone of an effective anti-acne program is learning to cleanse without moving bacteria across the face. The second is to know when to stop using anti-acne medications—those harsh, drying agents an adult cannot slather on forever without risking wrinkles and skin dehydration. And that is why I recommend a combination of astringents and healing lotions to combat acne without overdrying, to soothe blemishes away without scarring.

## The il-Makiage Morning Program for Acne/Problem Skin

You will need a complexion bar or cleansing milk (formulated for your skin type, or a product that contains sulphur); an acne-clarifying lotion or astringent; and a gentle healing lotion (such as an oily-skin preparation that contains azulin).

Use a complexion bar or milky cleanser (preferably one that contains sulphur) to clean your face and promote healing, but spread cleanser across the face with cotton—not fingers—to avoid spreading bacteria from forehead to cheeks to chin. Cleanse thoroughly twice to make sure skin is really clean.

Run astringent over your face to pick up the last traces of cleanser and to close pores. Repeat with fresh cotton until no oil or grime appears on the pad.

Putting makeup directly over blemishes only inflames them further. Use a healing lotion instead of a moisturizer. It will soothe your skin and act as your makeup base.

To reduce oiliness, use a water-based makeup. Apply it with a makeup sponge that you've washed in soap and water and sterilized in rubbing alcohol.

## The il-Makiage Evening Program for Acne/Problem Skin

Gently remove your makeup with cleansing milk, using cotton to apply the lotion to your face. Cleanse twice to make sure your face is really clean.

Wash your face with a complexion bar and water. Then use an astringent.

If you are past your teens, use an eye and throat cream occasionally even if it is too rich to leave on overnight. Despite what is happening to the rest of your face, those dry lines around eyes are getting drier all the time.

## Special Treatments for Acne/Problem Skin

Once a week, give yourself a mini-facial as described on pages 170 to 172, but forego the scrub—it will spread blemishes. Instead, wash with warm water to open your pores before you use your mask.

clay mask is perfect for troubled skin, but your complexion will benefit from the effects of any hardening mask. Leave your clay, mint, or other herbal mask on for fifteen minutes before removing it with cotton. Then apply astringent to close and tighten the pores.

## If You Break Out

You won't break out nearly so often if you follow the proper skin-care regime. But when you do, think of it as a temporary setback.

It's hard to wait for blemishes to disappear, but a hands-off policy is the only way to deal with breakouts. Pick at a pimple and it may erupt into a boil; squeeze it and you increase the chances of permanent scarring. Keep fingers away and the blemish will heal itself quickly. To help it along, dip a cotton swab in clarifying lotion and dab it gently on the blemish several times a day.

After your teens, it is unwise to put drying lotions all over your face; your problem could be compounded by patches of dry skin. If you see signs of surface dehydration—like taut epidermal skin with deep blemishes beneath—use a moisturizer for oily skin to normalize the affected areas.

## Acne After Twenty-Five

Repeated acne attacks after your early twenties demand the attention of a dermatologist. You may be allergic to something in your environment, or your problem could be the result of a hormonal imbalance. Above all, don't irritate a late-blooming attack of acne. I have seen terrible post-acne scars on women whose older skin was extremely sensitive.

# SPECIAL TREATMENTS

## Skin Scrubs

Exfoliants, "peels," or skin scrubs speed up the skin's shedding of dead cells and surface debris, revitalize circulation, and replace dull, flaky surface skin with a fresh, clean glow. The regular use of exfoliants will help your skin look and function better, leaving it brighter, cleaner, healthier.

Anyone can use a skin scrub *except* those with acne/problem skin or dry and sensitive skin. Slough once a week if you have dry skin; once or twice a week if skin is mixed; every other day if skin is oily, and your complexion will bloom.

### The Types of Sloughers

Exfoliants come in several different forms:

The washcloth has been used as a scrub for generations. Rubbing lightly with a damp washcloth, working in small circles over cheeks and forehead, is a simple way to slough off those dead cells that dull the skin's surface. But because the washcloth can "burn" the skin, it should only be used as an *occasional* alternative to a skin scrub—and never by women with sensitive skin.

So-called peels are applied wet. When they set on the skin, they are rubbed off, taking dead cells and debris with them.

Exfoliating sponges are fibrous, abrasive pads that may contain soap. Although they're very popular, these sponges are rough and tough on the skin. Use only with a very light touch.

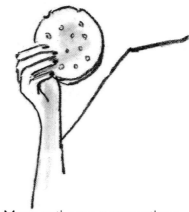

Many anti-acne preparations speed up the rate at which skin cells are shed. They are effective "invisible exfoliants" for those with acne/problem skin.

I prefer a creamy, "botanical" skin scrub (one made from organic materials) for safe, thorough exfoliation. Since you massage these creamy scrubs into your skin with your own hands, there is virtually no way of injuring your skin using one of these sloughers.

Choose natural exfoliators to rev up your tired complexion—or make your own scrub using natural ingredients from your own kitchen.

**A gentle scrub.** Blend two parts sugar to one part honey to form a paste. Thin with a few drops of water if the mixture seems too rich for your complexion.

**A hardworking scrub.** For a slightly more abrasive slougher, blend two parts *very finely ground* almonds to one part honey to form a paste.

To give skin a clearer, whiter appearance, add a dash of lemon juice to either of the above scrubs. The sugar or honey will neutralize the acidic citrus juice, minimizing drying, while the lemon juice works to "lift" the color of the skin.

### Using a Scrub

Skin scrubs have a much more abrasive texture than other skin-care products and must be softened with water before application. Before using a scrub, let the steam from a bath or shower open your pores and leave your skin soft and hydrated.

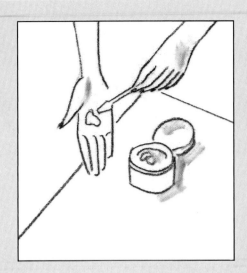

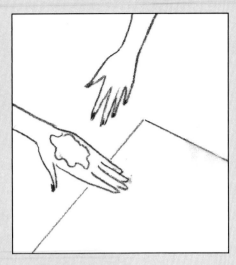

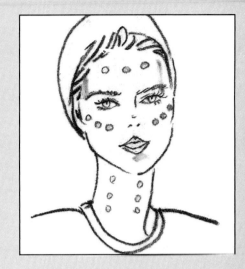

**1.** Scoop out a teaspoonful of scrub and place it in the palm of your wet hand.

**2.** Dip your other hand in water and mix the scrub until you can work with it easily.

**3.** Apply the scrub to the face and neck in a three-dot pattern.

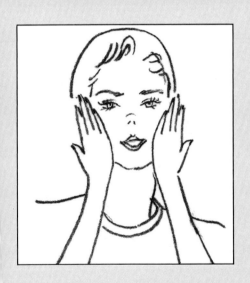

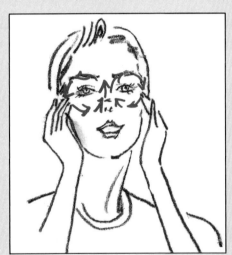

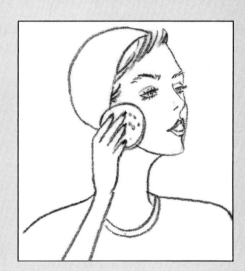

**4.** With your palms open, massage the scrub into cheeks, chin, and jawline using an upward circular motion. Continue for at least a minute so that the skin is cleansed deep down. Using the middle fingers of both hands, lightly scrub above the mouth. Scrub forehead in a side-to-side motion as if you were using a cleanser.

**5.** Massage *very gently* in a wide circle around the eyes and continue by gently cleansing the sides of the nose and around the nostrils. Scrub the neck clean, using the two-finger technique in upward, circular motions, beginning at the base of the neck and ending at the jawline.

**6.** Standing at the sink or in the shower, sponge off the scrub, beginning at the neck and working up. Work gently, especially in delicate skin areas. Rinse off excess scrub with lukewarm water.

## Scrub with Caution

Even natural scrubs can be over-used. If you have normal or dry skin, limit your exfoliating to once or twice a week; and no matter what your skin type, don't scrub daily. Too much of even a good thing is too much for your skin.

Beware of so-called "organic scrubs" that contain silica. It's a known skin irritant.

If your skin is sensitive, keep scrubbing particularly gentle. Apricot scrubs may scratch; others may contain additives that cause rashes or broken capillaries. Search for an especially gentle product or try my honey/sugar scrub: The sugar dissolves as you use it, making overuse impossible.

If scrubbing spreads blemishes on your oily skin, stop! Use a soothing mask instead to revive your complexion.

# THE ONCE-A-WEEK TWENTY-MINUTE MINIFACIAL

The mask is at the heart of the once-a-week minifacial treatment. Facial masks are roughly divided into two categories: *hardening* masks that cling to the surface of the skin to soak up excess oil and lift off dirt and debris, and *nourishing masks* that penetrate tired, dry skin to moisturize and revitalize it.

Check the condition of your pores and review the results of your blotter test before choosing a mask. If you have tight, small pores and dry skin, you need a moisturizing mask; if you have large pores, a hardening mask will benefit you most.

Deep-cleansing clay masks are the ultimate in hardening masks, and the ultimate in combating excess oil and soothing acne/problem skin.

For oily but unblemished skin, a mint mask is a cool, refreshing clarifier. Or try a homemade henna mask to soak up excess moisture yet leave the skin dewy:

Mix one tablespoon natural colorless henna with enough warm water to form a paste. Moisten gauze strips and spread gauze over forehead, cheeks, chin, and nose. Apply the mask over the gauze spread and allow to dry for about fifteen minutes.

If you have exceptionally dry or relatively mature skin (thirty-five or over), choose a nourishing mask that contains collagen or added vitamins. Or treat yourself to this homemade deepmoisturizing mask: Mix two whole eggs with five teaspoons of olive oil and ¼ teaspoon of honey. Stir well and apply to dry areas of your face.

## A Salon-Quality Minifacial

### Step One: Presteaming the Skin

While constant steam heat can cause the skin to sag, briefly steaming the face before your minifacial softens the surface of the skin, opens clogged pores, and makes it easier for your mask to lift away dirt and penetrate deeply. If you have time, sit in a bath or stand in the shower until your skin is baby-soft; then begin your facial.

Or fill a basin with steaming water, bend low over the water, and tent your head with a towel to trap steam near your face. (If it's uncomfortable for you to breathe, you are too close to the water! Stand back and let the steam work gently.) If time is at a premium, simply swathe your face with a warm, moist towel for a few minutes until heat has penetrated the skin.

How long should you steam? No more than three minutes if your skin is sensitive and never more than ten, even if your complexion is oily.

## Step Two:
## Preliminary Cleansing

First, use a milky cleanser, then thoroughly refresh your face with tonic or clarifying lotion. Finally, use a skin scrub to exfoliate dirt and debris.

## Step Three:
## Applying the Mask

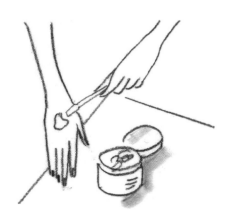

Put a few tablespoonsful of mask onto the back of one hand.

Using two fingers, apply the mask in short, even upward strokes. If you are using a hardening mask, work from the jawline up—you don't want to dry out the sensitive skin on your neck. If you are using a nourishing mask, work from the base of the neck up. And always leave a large circle around each eye free of the mask.

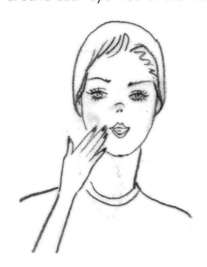

## Step Four:
## Eye and Throat Cream

If you have left your neck free of the mask, massage eye and throat cream into it. Then soak two pieces of cotton in cold water, place them over your closed eyelids, and relax.

## Step Five:
## Removing the Mask

After ten to fifteen minutes, remove the cotton eye pads and begin removing the mask.

To soften a hardening mask, moisten three long strips of cotton and wring out excess water. Lie down. Now lay one strip of cotton across your chin and along your jawline; lay the second across your nose and cheeks; and position the third across your forehead. Let the mask absorb the water and soon you will feel it begin to loosen. Now wipe each area with the moist cotton strips you used to loosen the mask; clean first along chin and jawline, next across cheeks and nose, and, last, across your forehead. Then wipe away any remaining mask with a fresh cotton strip or soft facial sponge.

**Important note:** Never leave a hardening mask on your face for more than fifteen minutes; it will start to irritate the skin, leaving you with temporary but annoying red marks on your face.

Nourishing masks are quite easy to remove. After ten or fifteen minutes, most of the mask solution has penetrated into the skin. Simply take a moist facial sponge and wipe away the excess. Then blot your face with a towel and follow with a moisturizer to counteract the drying effects of the water.

**A mask for mixed skin.** Apply a mint mask or some other hardening mask over the oily T-zone. Then fill in drier areas with a nourishing mask.

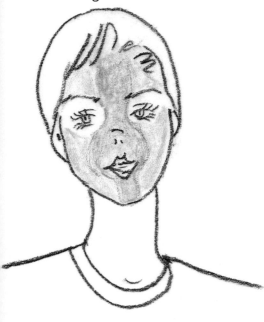

## After the Mask

You can apply makeup with no ill effects right after you've removed your mask. Although I usually do the minifacial at night, I often use a mask before a speaking engagement or television appearance, then apply my moisturizer and foundation as usual. My skin's renewed vitality is a visible, healthy luster that glows right through my makeup.

# TAKING CARE OF FACIAL HAIR

Even a small growth of facial hair—above the lip, on the chin, on the cheek—can spoil the look of the beautiful complexion you've worked so hard to attain. But if facial hair is a very common problem, so is it very easy to rectify.

There are four standard methods for eliminating or masking unsightly facial hair: waxing, bleaching, electrolysis, and Depilatron. The first two can be done quickly and easily at home; the last two require a professional's help.

**Waxing** is a great option for removing a very light fuzz of hair—but only for those women whose skin can stand up to some tugging. (Those with sensitive skin or an appreciable amount of facial hair should seek other alternatives—waxing encourages thicker hair growth and can cause a rash.)

Waxing is very easy to do at home with a commercially prepared kit. First, heat the wax over a very low flame until it reaches the consistency of chewing gum, then brush a very thin strip of wax over each side of the upper lip in the direction of the hair growth. Press down on the strip with your fingers, wait a few seconds, then gently peel off the wax (in the direction opposite the application) while holding skin down

with your other hand. Immediately place fingers over the area to stop minor stinging. Then, with a cotton ball, sweep a solution of borax and water over the area to keep it free from rashes.

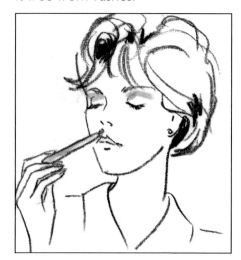

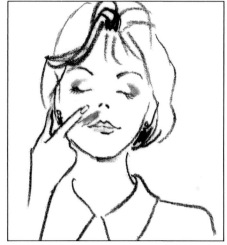

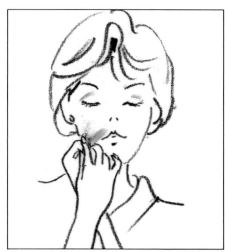

**Bleaching** doesn't get rid of hair, but it's ideal for hiding a fine, light growth, particularly above the lip or on the sides of the face. Buy a commercially prepared bleaching kit at any drugstore—but be sure to do a patch test before applying it extensively.

Mix two parts developer to one part bleach (or follow package directions), then smooth mixture on the hair you want to fade. Leave on for about five minutes before removing with a washcloth.

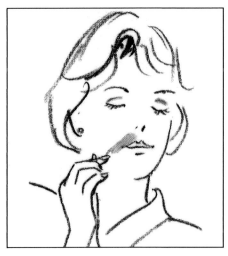

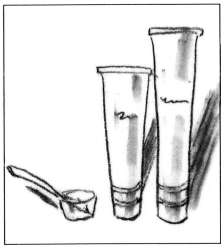

You can also lighten your brows at home with facial hair bleach. Since you want brows that are the same color or a scant shade lighter than your hair color, make sure you don't overbleach.

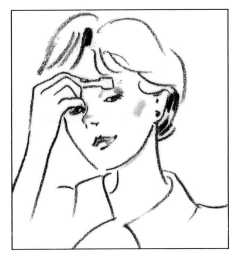

Smooth the mixture against the direction of hair growth for an even application. Bleach works fast, so start checking the color by lifting a few hairs with a small spatula within sixty seconds after application. If the ends are lighter than the center, reapply over darker hairs.

**Electrolysis** and **Depilatron** are both methods of permanent hair removal that can only be done by trained professionals. The end result of both techniques is the same—but the methods of getting there are very different.

Electrolysis involves the insertion of a small electric needle through the pores, under the skin, and into the hair follicles, killing the roots of the hair. Because it attacks hair growth at its source, it is faster but more painful than Depilatron.

Depilatron is a permanent method of hair removal using an electric tweezer to send currents through the hair and into the papilla, the white gel that holds the hair firmly in place. When the papilla dries, hair slips out easily. This process is painless but time-consuming. After a few sessions, softer hair growth is noticeable; eventually the hair follicle is destroyed and hair ceases to grow.

If you choose to have facial hair removed permanently, be sure to have it done by a reputable professional at a salon. Ask your hairstylist, cosmetologist, or friends for recommendations.

# SKIN PROTECTION FOR ALL SEASONS

We all know that our skin is affected by the weather. In a four-season climate, it will bloom in the spring and fall, when conditions are neither hot and humid nor very cold and dry. In summer and winter, however, even the best of complexions can wilt and wither.

Because both heat and cold steal moisture from your skin, your skin must be prepared to counteract the adverse effects of extreme weather well before the heat is on or the snow begins to fly.

## Your Winter Protection Plan

No matter what your skin type, the key to winterizing your complexion is scrupulous moisturizing. Even if you have oily skin with enough natural moisture to protect you from the effects of wind and cold, your surface skin can become dry, chapped, and temporarily dehydrated. If your skin tends to become extremely dry in winter, use a thick day cream instead of your usual light liquid moisturizer; it will give you all the extra protection you need to survive those blusters and squalls.

Lips dry out first, so put lip balm under lipstick or gloss and carry it at all times to reapply as needed. Massage a little eye and throat cream along the lip line and you'll prevent dry skin lines from developing.

Winter sunlight can burn, especially in combination with wind. Smooth on sunscreen whenever you expect to be out in the winter sun for any length of time. If you are skating outdoors, skiing, or heading for a snowy resort, remember that high altitudes intensify the damaging effects of ultraviolet radiation. (Snow reflects glare even more effectively than a sandy beach!) Protect your eyes with sunglasses or, better yet, goggles. Apply a sunblock over exposed areas and massage eye and throat cream around your eyes and on your neck. And because sun and snow together are so dehydrating, add an extra layer of moisturizer over your sunscreen.

## Spring and Fall Skin Strategies

As the snow melts or the leaves turn bright, spend a few minutes examining your skin. If it's dry, flaky, or generally dehydrated, use a skin scrub to get rid of superficial dry patches and give healthy undersurface skin a chance to rise to the surface. And celebrate the coming of the new season with a minifacial or thorough moisturizing massage.

## Your Summer Protection Plan

Depending on your skin type and the type of heat you encounter during the summer, your skin may need more or less moisturizing protection now than during more temperate times of the year.

If summer in your area means blistering heat and high humidity, you may need to stop moisturizing the T-zone while the weather is steamy. Concentrate instead on keeping hypersensitive and drier areas (like the delicate skin around your eyes) protected. If necessary, daytime moisturizing can always be supplemented with a night cream.

Those with dry skin may find that even in the sultriest weather they still need extra protection to replenish the natural moisture lost to heat and perspiration. Smooth it on! Not only will moisturizing keep skin supple, but it will defend your complexion from the environmental pollutants that stick to skin in humid weather.

## Your Place in the Sun

For many people, summer means sun. But if you want your sun time to be fun time, it's important to follow some sensible precautions.

Sunshine is, in many ways, excellent for the skin. It's great for drying up acne and excess oiliness, and it speeds the turnover of new skin cells, making many summer complexions newer- and healthier-looking than in the bleak winter months. And you know how your skin glows when you have a tan!

There's no reason you can't enjoy the sun, but start slowly; go out early in the morning or late in the afternoon for your first exposures of the season. Then gradually extend the time you spend catching those rays. But never expose your skin unless you've slathered on the sunscreen.

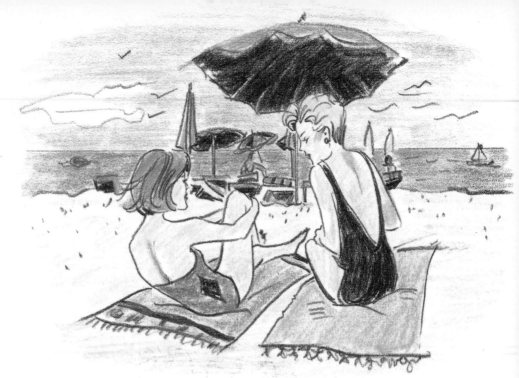

Apply lotion about half an hour before you head for the beach and you'll get that healthy glow— not a painful, drying burn.

The protective ingredients in sunscreen wash off in water, so reapply it generously every time you step out of the ocean or pool. (Chlorinated water, in particular, is very drying to the skin.

Besides reapplying sunscreen, be sure to moisturize your entire body after you shower.) On very hot days you will need to reapply sunscreen quite frequently, as much of it will be washed away by your own perspiration.

As you get older, your skin gets drier, more prone to discoloration and more apt to burn. From your late twenties on, prudence dictates avoiding direct exposure to the sun as much as possible. Put on eye cream before you go out into the bright sunlight, and when you're out, wear a hat and sunglasses as well as a sunscreen.

## Skin in Transit

For the luckiest among us, summertime means vacation time! But no matter what season you do your jet-setting, plane travel can be so dehydrating that by the end of a six-hour flight you may feel as though your skin has aged twenty years!

Here's my solution: Don't wear any foundation when you get on the plane. Instead, massage in moisturizer periodically throughout the flight. Then, half an hour before landing, head for the rest room and give yourself a final application of moisturizer, then a touch of makeup. When you reach your destination, your skin will be smooth and moisturized and your makeup fresh. Happy landings!

# CHAPTER THREE

# YOUR SKIN CYCLE

Every woman feels changes in her mood, energy level, and sense of physical well-being at different times of the month. And even the briefest glance in the mirror tells us that skin color, condition, and texture also vary perceptibly under the influence of the hormones that control menstruation. But just as understanding how those hormonal swings affect your body can help you stay active throughout your menstrual cycle, so can it help you to keep your skin "in the pink"—healthy and glowing—no matter what the time of the month.

# 28-Day Skin Cycle

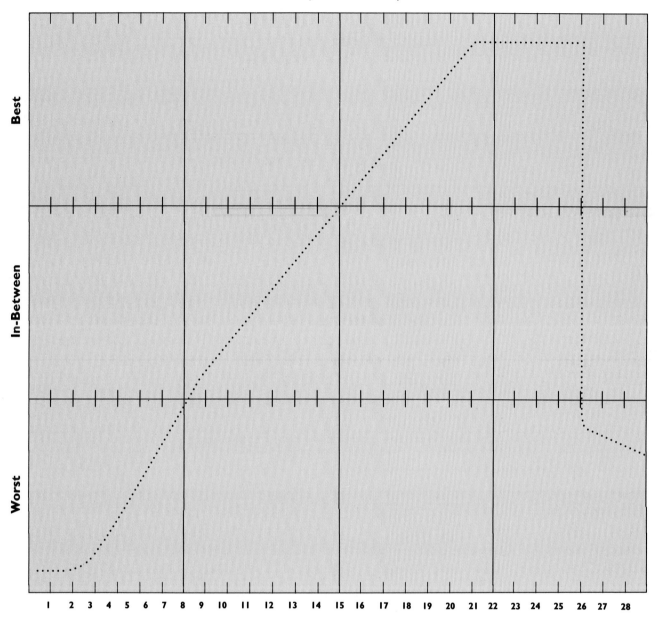

Here is a graph of the condition of your skin at various times during an average twenty-eight-day cycle, along with indications for the best times of the month to give your skin special treatment. Some women have shorter or longer cycles, so adjust the graph to reflect *your* skin cycle precisely.

# THE BEST TIME

In the middle of your cycle, generally starting about the eighteenth day of a twenty-eight-day cycle and continuing for about a week, the condition of your complexion is at its best. No matter what your skin type, pores are tighter, blemishes fewer; skin feels smoother and cleaner than at any other time of the month and radiates a healthy glow.

# THE WORST TIME

Anyone who has ever woken up with a premenstrual attack of acne or rough, dry, flaking skin can readily attest to the fact that the least desirable skin characteristics are generally exaggerated toward the beginning of your menstrual period. Many women have only to look in the mirror to tell how soon their period will begin: Skin becomes pale, sallow, drained of color; pores become visible to the naked eye (and open to impurities); oily skins become unmanageably slick; and dry complexions wither.

Every woman's complexion has its own way of reacting to the slight temperature elevation, fluid retention, and other changes that presage menstruation. What about yours?

If you have normal, combination, or oily skin, your skin is oilier than usual; more acid flows to the skin surface through larger pores. Blemishes are more likely to erupt, as well. Your skin loses its healthy color and darker, more prominent circles may appear under your eyes. And hormones can trigger an even more permanent beauty problem, as well: an increase in the growth of facial hair.

If you have a dry complexion, your skin will either suddenly be rife with excess oils or your normally small pores may close up tight. Your skin feels rough; it may even flake or become dehydrated. Broken capillaries may become more pronounced, and skin color—either sallowed or reddened by the hormonal flux—will be at its worst.

# THE IN-BETWEEN TIME

While you can expect your skin's tone, texture, and condition to change abruptly—even overnight—as you approach your menstrual period, during the two weeks between the extremes of your monthly skin cycle the improvement in your skin is slow and steady. But with just a little extra care, as well as some cooperation from nature, you can help to accelerate the regeneration process and look your best every day of the month.

# **Y**OUR SKIN-CYCLE PROGRAM

An effective skin-cycle program is one that helps you balance bad skin days, makes the most of great skin days, and allows your complexion to glow most of the time in between.

An ounce of prevention is worth a pound of cure—and the first basic component of making your skin-cycle program work for you is *knowledge*. For one month, redo the skin-type analysis *every week* and jot the results in your notebook. Learning how hormonal fluctuations affect each zone of your face will prepare you to anticipate and offset the less-than-beautiful side effects of Mother Nature's handiwork. You'll be ready and able to stop problems before they start—and since complexion woes (particularly acne and broken capillaries) that begin during the menstrual cycle *can* endure long after the critical week has passed, to be fore-warned is to be forearmed!

Once you have established precisely which changes you can expect during your monthly skin cycle, it's time to put the second component of the program into action—by beginning to use harder-working formulations of your usual skin products to combat the problems that crop up at various times of the month. If you have dry or mixed skin, for example, you may find that your complexion becomes 1-zone oily when you menstruate. Using a tonic with a minimum of alcohol is a skin-saver while your complexion regenerates during the three weeks between each period, since too much alcohol can strip your already tight, dry skin. But in the days just before your period and continuing through that hormonally difficult week, you'll need a tonic with a higher concentration of alcohol to control that oily shine. Then, on the second day of your menstrual doldrums, give yourself a minifacial using two masks—a moisture-rich formulation on cheeks and a hardening mask on forehead, nose, and chin, and you'll boost your skin's ability to regain its natural balance.

The third principal component of the skin-cycle program has to do with the special treatments that can nourish and balance your skin while hormonal levels rise and fall. When your skin is in its best shape, at the midpoint of your cycle, it's sufficient to moisturize and cleanse it. If you're past your twenties and your skin needs revitalizing, your good skin days are the best days to treat your skin to collagen.

But at the worst time of the month, pamper your skin with a facial to rev up texture and tone.

And in the in-between time, exfoliate—scrub away the dead outer layers to help your skin regenerate itself and make it glow.

# **R**EADY, SET—GLOW!

Is there anything you can do to give your personalized skin-cycle program a beauty boost to minimize the effects of raging hormones? You bet there is! In the week preceding the onset of your period, make just three adjustments to your usual skin-care regime and skin will *normalize* itself—and you'll sail through even your "worst" complexion days looking your best!

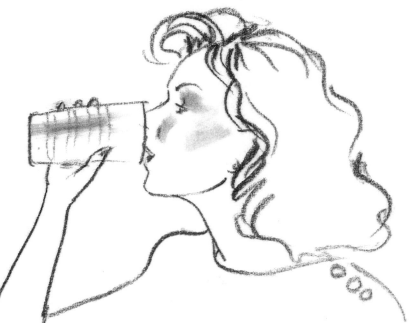

**1. Drink six to eight glasses of water every day.** If you've been bypassing this natural clarifier, you've overlooked the key factor in keeping your skin functioning at its peak. Kick off your skin-cycle program by giving your thirsty complexion the refreshment it needs most and you'll see a marked improvement in the condition of your skin within days.

**2. Exfoliate.** Step up your scrub-and-mask regime in the days just before your period and you'll sail into your bad complexion days with fresher, healthier skin. And you may stop skin problems before they start.

**3. Moisturize, moisturize, moisturize!** Drinking lots of water and exfoliating regularly (but never *every* day!) brings new skin cells to the surface. Moisturizer will protect the effects of skin regeneration and help fresh skin to help itself fend off any hormonally caused dryness.

Just these small changes in your usual skin-care program will bring about big changes: Skin will be clearer, cleaner—even the color of your complexion will bloom. To maximize those beauty benefits, get plenty of sleep, cut your alcohol consumption, and *stop smoking.* Your skin cleans itself while you snooze; get too little sleep and you deny your complexion the time it needs to rid

## Color and Your Skin Cycle

**S**ince your skin is drained of color around the time of your period, why not add more color to your makeup? First, use a toner to counteract any sallowness. Then, bring on the bright blushes, shadows, and lip colors to counteract that tired, drawn look.

itself of impurities. Drinking and smoking dehydrate skin and may even sallow the rosy tone that drinking plenty of water can impart.

Watch your diet: If at all possible, avoid eating pork and shellfish in the critical days before the onset of menstruation. Pork fat is especially difficult for the cells to break down—and shellfish, which releases toxins into the body, takes three days to fully digest. These foods may tantalize the tastebuds, but their effects can show up on your face *days* after you've eaten them.

And finally, put your skin-care program into high gear by making these skin-cycle tips part of your daily regime.

# THE IL-MAKIAGE SKIN-CYCLE PROGRAM FOR DRY OR SENSITIVE SKIN

The luckiest of sensitive-skinned beauties report no changes during the menstrual week—they can continue their usual skin-care regime and spot-treat drier patches with emollient creams as needed.

But if your complexion becomes noticeably oilier, or even breaks out, finish your nightly cleansing with an alcohol-free tonic to close pores and restore the skin's protective acid mantle; then eliminate your nighttime moisturizer to allow your skin to breathe.

Despite your skin's sudden oiliness, stay away from harsh scrubs that can scratch the skin or break capillaries. Instead, rinse the skin more thoroughly than usual after cleansing to gently deep-clean your hypersensitive complexion.

Rich emollient masks, usually a mainstay of your poreless complexion, may only compound the excess oiliness that plagues you during your period. Use the following naturally moisturizing, nonacidic homemade mask, instead, to balance excessive oiliness without dehydrating your normally dry skin. This refresher not only helps heal blemishes and softens skin but even soothes undereye puffiness.

**Cucumber mask:** Peel and shred one cucumber. Mix with honey to form a paste and apply to clean face. Leave on fifteen to twenty minutes, then rinse off with lukewarm water.

**Other treatments:** Treat your skin to a vitamin ampule—or even a seven-night ampule sequence—during your "bad skin" week, and your complexion will glow! Vitamins A, D, and E stimulate the metabolism of the skin, helping it to regenerate and normalize faster. Smooth the vitamin-rich ampule treatment from the base of the neck up; then, to speed penetration, cover the area with a warm, moist towel for no more than three minutes. (Steam can redden sensitive skin for *hours*.)

# THE IL-MAKIAGE SKIN-CYCLE PROGRAM FOR DEMANDING SKIN

If your skin becomes flaky during the week of menstruation, and if your "pinch test" reveals that your natural collagen fibers are breaking down, you have demanding skin—skin that needs not only added nourishment but extra help to stay at its firmest.

To give your skin's substructure an added boost, your skin-care products should all be collagen-enriched: Use a milky-cleanser with added collagen to deep-clean and nourish; then follow with a collagen tonic to restore the acid mantle. Choose collagen moisturizers to protect natural fibers from the effects of heat and cold, then alternate between a rich moisture cream and a collagen cream as a nighttime treat. Scrub away dead cells and debris gently—but, to keep skin bright, clear, and sufficiently moist, no more than twice a month.

During the week of your period, demanding skin can wither; head for the salon *every other month* for a revitalizing paraffin mask. (Warm masks, when repeated too often, can cause capillaries to break.) And in between, treat yourself to these homemade masks to banish flaky patches and nourish the skin.

**Avocado mask:** Peel and pit one ripe avocado, then mash well with a fork. Blend in enough honey to form a paste and apply to face. Relax for ten to fifteen minutes, then remove with a facial sponge or moist cotton.

**Normalizing mask:** Separate one egg. Mix the yolk with five drops of olive oil and ¼ teaspoon of honey. Blend well, then apply to driest portions of your face (usually cheeks) to eliminate flaking skin. Then, blend the egg white with five drops of lemon juice and apply to nose to control oiliness.

Rinse off with clear water after ten to fifteen minutes.

**Other treatments:** Vaporize your bedroom to boost your complexion's ability to breathe in moisture. If your skin is oily, use a cold-air vaporizer; if dry, opt for a warm-air vaporizer instead.

Demanding skin will bloom straight through the menstrual week if a seven-night collagen ampule sequence is substituted for night cream. And at least once during your bad skin week use a nourishing mask to counteract hormonally rooted dryness.

# THE IL-MAKIAGE SKIN-CYCLE PROGRAM FOR MIXED OR NORMAL-TO-DRY SKIN

During the menstrual week, mixed skins shine with excess moisture and even normal-to-dry skin can develop T-zone oiliness. Though it is a temptation to fight oily break-through with harsh drying agents, alcohol, benzoyl peroxide, and sulphur can dehydrate surface skin, trapping oil and sebum beneath.

Use a milky cleanser formulated for mixed skins to deep-clean without drying; then spot-treat oilier areas with tonic until skin regains its natural balance. Forego a nighttime moisturizer to allow skin to breathe (your natural oils during the menstrual week will sufficiently nourish the skin), but always use an eye cream. Your T-zone may seem unmanageably oily, but delicate undereye skin cannot produce enough oil to protect itself from the elements.

Boost regeneration by scrubbing gently with a slougher after your skin has been softened by a warm bath or shower. Then treat skin to a creamy mask for mixed skin at least once during your bad skin week—or try the homemade Normalizing Mask to moisten dry areas while controlling oil on the T-zone.

**Other treatments:** Particularly in winter, hydrate your skin with a mist vaporizer filled with mineral water.

# THE IL-MAKIAGE SKIN-CYCLE PROGRAM FOR NORMAL-TO-OILY SKIN

Nothing turns normally controllably oily skin to problem skin like the menstrual week! When hormones fluctuate, pores open and oil flows; skin becomes greasy, sallow, and, worst of all, blemished.

Yet by treating your skin with products that are meant to dry, you may be stimulating oil glands to work harder, compounding your difficulty rather than relieving it. Surface skin dehydrates, trapping oil beneath the skin, where large blemishes begin. During your menstrual week, you must cleanse more often—not more harshly—to keep surface skin clean yet supple enough to rid itself of excess moisture. Use a soapless soap and a tonic with 10 percent alcohol as part of your morning and evening regime; then refresh with an alcohol-free tonic throughout the day to control oiliness without overdrying. A medicated nighttime emulsion will help heal blemishes while you sleep throughout your bad skin days; but as soon as excessive oiliness subsides, opt for an emulsion that contains azulin to normalize without dehydrating.

Keep any anti-acne medications or normalizers away from the delicate undereye skin. And don't forget the eye cream—no matter what is going on in the rest of your face, this fragile skin needs extra moisture throughout your skin cycle.

Scrub no more often than every other day with a slougher to speed up skin regeneration—then treat yourself to a hardening mask to deep-clean, soothe blemishes, and drink up excess oil.

**Other treatments:** In spring and summer, wear a tinted moisturizer rather than a foundation to help skin breathe while protecting it from pollution and heat.

# THE IL-MAKIAGE SKIN-CYCLE PROGRAM FOR ACNE/PROBLEM SKIN

Acne/problem skin is the most discouraging skin type under the best of circumstances, and during the week of your period it may become overwhelming. Skin sallows, making your complexion appear lifeless and dull. Meanwhile, pores open wide, allowing unmanageable amounts of oil to flow to the skin's surface—and exposing your complexion to a barrage of external impurities that can encourage blemishes to flourish. Yet acne/problem skin is often sensitive skin, as well. Caustic drying agents can only compound the situation, making skin surface taut and sealing oil deep within the dermis, where large blemishes and cysts develop. While the temptation to dry your skin to the point of peeling may be hard to resist, the only way to maintain this type of skin, promote healing, and encourage normalization is to go with the flow—to allow excess oils passage out of the dermis—and to keep the surface of the skin scrupulously clean.

Drink *a minimum* of six to eight glasses of water every day of your menstrual week to moisturize internally while promoting cell regeneration. If you have been dehydrating the surface of your skin with harsh chemicals and drying agents formulated for teenage skin, undo the damage by following this simple regime until surface skin has lost its taut, dry appearance: Cleanse morning and evening with a milky cleanser, then tone with an alcohol-free tonic. And once a day, nourish the skin with this simple homemade mask.

**Yogurt normalizer:** Mix two to three teaspoons of plain yogurt with ½ teaspoon of sugar. Blend well, then apply to dry, taut areas of the face. Rinse off after fifteen minutes.

**183**

Once skin regains its balance and is supple enough to allow subsequent treatments to penetrate and natural oils to flow, begin this gentle regime to heal blemished skin without dehydrating.

Cleanse morning and evening with a soapless soap, then deep-clean with a 10 percent alcohol tonic. Keep a small bottle of tonic—or a mineral water spritzer—on hand all day long to refresh your skin and counteract oily shine. You may wish to use an anti-acne clarifying lotion, as well, but be sure to apply it only to blemished areas. (Oily skin is *not* wrinkle-proof!) And whether you're treating yourself to tonic, clarifier, or removing your cleanser, use only 100 percent cotton. Manmade "cosmetic puffs" can irritate your skin and inflame blemishes.

Because exfoliating scrubs or sloughers can spread blemishes from one area of the face to another, never use these products on acne/problem skin. Instead, treat your complexion to a hardening mask to remove debris and control excess oil twice during the week of your period. And be sure to follow up with a nighttime emulsion that contains azulin to encourage healing.

Because oil from skin and hair can collect on pillowcases, sometimes reinfecting clear areas with bacteria, change your pillowcases every day. Then wash them in a mild soap—detergents, too, are irritating to problem skin.

And during the week of your menstrual period, avoid makeup as much as possible. But to keep oil from breaking through your foundation when makeup is absolutely necessary, give yourself a tightening mask first—then go over your face with an ice cube to close pores.

**Special treatments.** Vitamin A, applied topically, can regenerate the cells and speed exfoliation. Your dermatologist can recommend the right vitamin cream or lotion.

A sulphur mask can help acne to heal. Apply to blemished areas *only*, then rinse off after fifteen minutes.

# Extra Care for Tired Complexions

When you are finally "free" of the monthly hormonal fluctuations that regulate menstruation, your skin may need more help than ever!

Although tending to your skin with a gentle yet hardworking skin-care regime will help you always to look younger than your years, skin ages—and the substructure of the dermis can break down. Eventually almost every woman needs something extra to boost tired-looking skin.

The number of competing skin-care products is unbelievable; and what's even more unbelievable is that they all promise the fountain of youth. No product, no matter how exotic or costly, can make miracles, but a good product will temporarily plump up cells, smooth wrinkles, and protect the skin from the ravaging effects of wind and weather.

## Treatment Creams

Once your skin becomes very dry or tired-looking, you can use creams that contain extra-rich nourishing ingredients as well as moisturizing agents.

I prefer treatment creams that combine plant-derived oils with added vitamins. Vitamins A and B are reputed to have a healing and nourishing effect on the skin; Vitamin E cream can be particularly vitalizing.

## Vitamin Ampules

Good things come in small packages! These little vials are packed with concentrated liquid vitamins that can revitalize even time-worn, overworked, and undernourished skin, regardless of calendar age. As single treatments, they are relatively expensive, but the effects of these powerful little vials can be well worth the investment.

To use vitamin ampules, gradually empty the contents of the vial into the palm of your hand, rub palms together, then pat onto clean skin. To supercharge the deep-down benefits, swathe your face with a warm, moist towel to increase the treatment's penetrating power.

Depending on the condition of your skin, ampules can be used on consecutive days or every other day. Most women find that a three-to-seven-day treatment series every two months is sufficient.

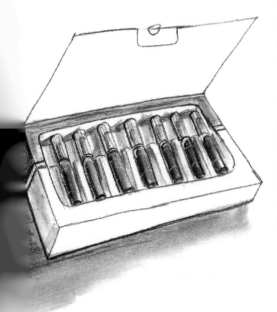

## Collagen

Collagen is probably *the* skin discovery of the last decade. The loss of the skin's natural elasticity is caused largely by the decline in internal sources of collagen. The theory behind collagen products is that when natural fibers are replaced by collagen from plant and animal sources, elasticity and skin tone return.

Many dermatologists replace collagen through a series of injections that literally shoot animal collagen into your skin. These injections temporarily smooth lines and wrinkles, and put new life back into the complexion. But the effect doesn't last more than three months.

Collagen-enriched creams and lotions put collagen back into the upper layer of skin, allowing it to temporarily look firmer. Use a collagen ampule and you will feel an immediate tightening of the skin tissues; best of all, the effect will last long enough so that if you use collagen on a daily basis for even one week you will reap definite visible results.

Once you've decided to try collagen, start with one or two products that contain it, then gradually change all of your skin-care products. Don't change skin-care routines; simply substitute firming, toning products for basic formulations.

But remember—you don't need collagen unless your skin is losing its firmness and tone. If you're in doubt, try the elasticity factor pinch test on page 153.

# Y OUR BODY SKIN CYCLE

Just as your facial skin reacts to the fluctuation of your hormones, so is your body skin sometimes oilier, sometimes drier, sometimes smooth, colorful, and firm—and sometimes in dire need of revitalization. During the oilier times of your cycle, try using your facial skin scrub as an allover body exfoliator. Afterward, smooth on body lotion for a wonderful two-stage body facial.

But when skin needs a little extra help, wash your troubles away in the most relaxing, revitalizing, convenient beauty spa of all—your bathtub.

# THE BATH— YOUR PERSONAL SPA

There is nothing like a nice, warm, up-to-your-neck bath for soaking away tension, encouraging relaxation, and just plain luxuriating—I love it! The bouyancy of water— the feeling of weightlessness it gives—is just right for making tension float away. And you can make your bath even more relaxing: When you first step into it, sit back, get comfortable; then inhale deeply through your nose and exhale through your mouth until you feel the muscles of your face, neck, and body relax completely. Bliss!

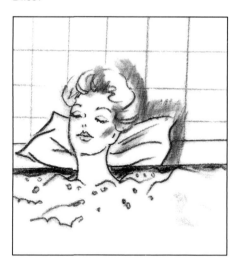

But your bath can be much more than a well-deserved respite from the stresses of everyday living. Oils, salts, and soaks can turn your tub into a beauty treatment that works hard to counteract the effects of your body skin cycle while you soak. Choose among these luxurious beauty boosters to eliminate any dryness, flaky skin, and excessive oiliness that surfaces during bad skin days, then follow up with a body mask (use the formula you find most effective for your complexion) on shoulders and chest to deep-clean problem areas. Skin will glow from head to toe!

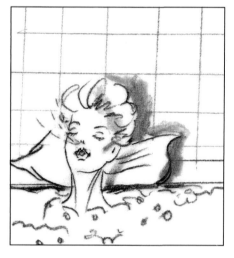

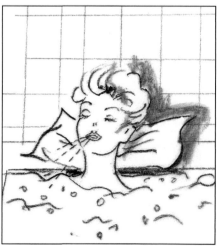

## Skin Cycle Soaks for Normal-to-Dry Skin

Flaking? Banish the thought! And banish that taut, dry feeling by soaking your skin problems away with your favorite bath oil.

Bath oils range in scent from flowery to woody to lemony, making your bath a heady experience. But do opt for a high-quality formulation. Chemically produced fragrances can irritate already-chapped skin, making you prone to rashes and breakouts. And less-expensive bath oils are often lanolin-based, leaving you (and your tub) with a greasy finish.

A little bath oil goes a long way—even a more expensive bath enhancer is economical when used in the recommended proportions. So shop for a bath oil scented only with pure botanical oils—your skin will thank you for it. And look for one that coats the skin with pure, processed oils. Not only will these emollients seal in moisture, but they will *penetrate* the skin, leaving your whole body smooth and refreshed.

## Skin Cycle Soaks for Normal-to-Oily Skin

**Henna** is not only a hair coloring and conditioner, it is also a wonderful treatment for oily skin. Add four cups of natural colorless henna to your bath to refresh skin, balance excess oil, and help heal blemishes. Or use it as a naturally gentle scrub *and* soak by adding as much as a kilo to your bath, then using the undissolved powder to exfoliate dead skin patches that spoil the smooth look and feel of oily skin. A quick shower will take off any residue, leaving skin polished and renewed, with a wonderful woodsy scent.

Another normalizer for oily skin: the **milk bath**. Add a quart of whole milk to your bath water, then settle back and enjoy! You'll step out of the tub with baby-soft—and well-balanced —skin.

## Revitalizing Baths for Every Body

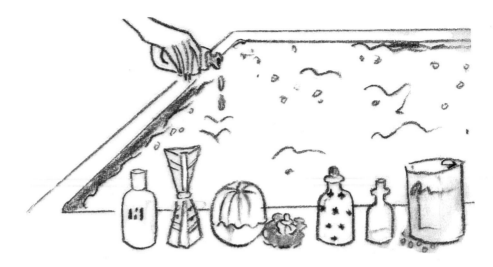

Because bath salts are natural softeners and gentle cleansers, they can be used to prepare any skin type to absorb moisturizing body lotion. Add **salts** to your bath and water stays clear and inviting; revel in a long, soothing soak and surface oils dissolve, leaving skin smooth, pores open.

Trying to clear out a head cold or put a particularly stressful day behind you? Add a few drops of **minty eucalyptus** oil to your tub. The wonderfully pungent pine scent relaxes and reenergizes— and since eucalyptus oil is available in most drug and health food stores, it is a great bath bargain.

## BODY LOTION MASSAGE

Be generous with your body lotion—as you pleasurably massage your "forgotten complexion," the skin of your body. For best results, always move your hands across your skin in a circular motion.

While standing, start by massaging lotion onto your arms; then proceed to your shoulders, the back of your neck, your breasts, your stomach, your behind, your back, and your upper thighs.

Sit down to massage feet, ankles, and calves. And finally, massage your hands (palm, back, and each finger). Your skin will be smooth, moist, and tingling all over.

# HEALTHY HAIR IS BEAUTIFUL HAIR

You can mousse it, gel it, even add highlights to spark some extra glow! Still, the best way to keep hair beautiful is to keep it healthy. Unless hair is shining, free of split ends, and alive with natural body, it cannot act as the ultimate accessory to your face—and can even be a detraction.

Maintaining the health of your hair is relatively simple if you maximize the positive, natural things you do to enhance it and minimize the negative effects of chemicals, the environment, stress, and diet. This isn't to say that you can never perm, artificially color, or blow-dry hair— you can have fun doing all those things if you take the time to offset the damage. So experiment—but temper those negative effects with some of these revitalizing treatments and you'll keep your crowning glory strong and glowing.

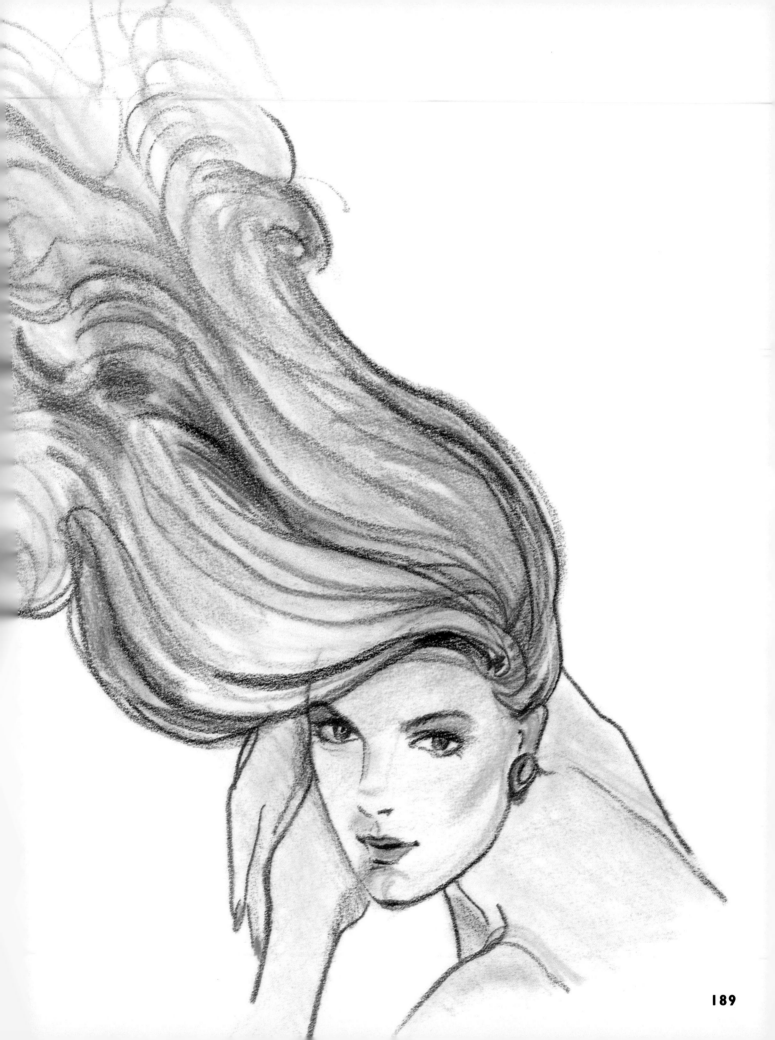

189

# SHAMPOO

Hair collects grime and dust fast, particularly if you live in a city. Yet, it is possible to overdo your shampooing, washing body and manageability right out of the hair and stripping its natural oils. If you wash your hair every day whether it needs it or not, your hair will certainly be clean, but it won't have the chance to replenish itself and shine with the natural proteins that come to the surface between shampoos. If your hair and scalp are very oily, you'll need to wash daily to rid hair of the excess oils that can raise havoc with your complexion (a henna shampoo can help control oiliness); but if your hair is dry and flyaway, if ends are split and ragged, and if your complexion is dry to normal, your overly scrupulous cleaning may be robbing your hair of the nutrients it needs to shine. Try shampooing only every other day for one week. If hair becomes more manageable, then less really is more for your hair's health—more kind, more gentle, and more natural.

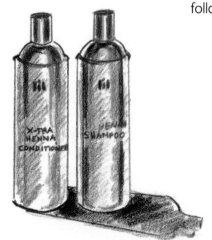

Remember the skin cycle? Your hair has a monthly cycle, too, tending to become drier or oilier and harder to manage just before your period. Switch shampoos at that time of the month to compensate for the changes in your hair; if you normally lather up with a shampoo for normal hair, choose a dry or oily formulation to adjust to hormonal fluctuations.

And whenever possible, avoid hair dryers; the blast of heat contributes to split ends. Instead, towel dry your hair until it stops dripping. Then run your hands through your hair to untangle it and allow it to dry naturally.

# CONDITION WITH HENNA

It's a good idea for all women to deep-condition their hair on occasion, but when you perm or color with chemicals, conditioning is a *must*. To counteract the effects of a perm or a harsh dye, I suggest a henna deep-conditioning treatment twenty-four hours later, and a follow-up ten days thereafter.

Other conditioners penetrate the hair shaft, moisturizing hair from within. But only henna actually *coats* the hair shaft to seal in natural moisture, increase shine, and keep protecting wash after wash.

Before you start, shampoo your hair and towel it dry. Then, working with both hands, massage conditioner all over the head, from scalp to ends. Comb through with a wide-tooth comb to distribute conditioner evenly; wrap hair with aluminum foil or a plastic bag, top with a warm towel (or heat cap), and leave in place for about twenty-five minutes. Remove the cap, rinse thoroughly, and comb out, starting at the ends to loosen tangles and to keep hair from tearing, and working up toward the scalp with longer strokes. Your conditioner keeps working long after you've rinsed it out, but to maximize those beneficial effects, avoid shampooing until the following day.

# **H**AIR MASSAGE

A quick hair massage helps strengthen roots, promote hair growth, and bolster circulation to the scalp.

Start at the nape or with the hair furthest from the crown. Grasp near roots and gradually work fingers toward the ends.

# **B**RUSHING

Proper brushing is *not* damaging to the hair; rather, it stimulates hair growth, strengthens the roots, thickens the hair, and makes it shine. To get the most out of your nightly brushing, put your head down when you brush, the more strokes the better (within reason and without stopping), in all directions.

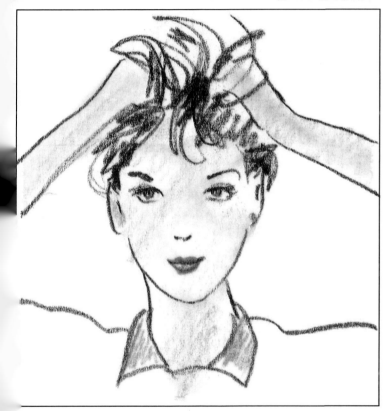

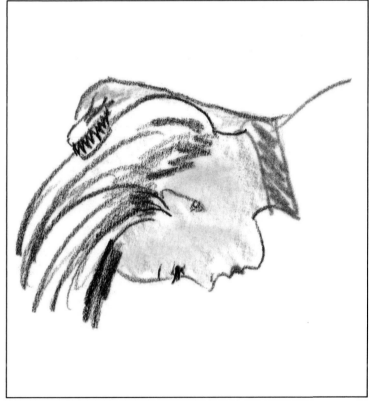

Tighten fingers around hair, pull gently, and slowly release. Work around your head until you reach the crown; then use both hands to grab and release, still working in a circle, with hands at a ninety-degree angle to each other.

Brushing can benefit permed, colored, or even damaged hair, as well. Just comb through first, working from the ends up toward the scalp, to remove tangles. And never brush wet hair; that kind of pulling and tearing *is* damaging.

# HENNA— THE NATURAL WAY TO HIGHLIGHT HAIR

Since the dawn of civilization, women have used henna to make themselves more beautiful. Cleopatra and the ladies of her court relied on it as a highlighter, a colorant, a healing conditioner, and a beautifying treatment. It is even mentioned in the Bible's Song of Songs, where Solomon sings of "a cluster of henna in the vineyards of En Gedi."

Why has henna endured as a beautifier all these many millenia? Simply because it is effective.

In an age of fads, with new products being introduced nearly every day, henna is the one colorant that withstands the test of time. And because it's a 100 percent natural product—a water-soluble powder made from the leaves, roots, and stems of the Lawsonia plant—henna works its magic without damaging, without drying, and without chemically altering the structure of the hair.

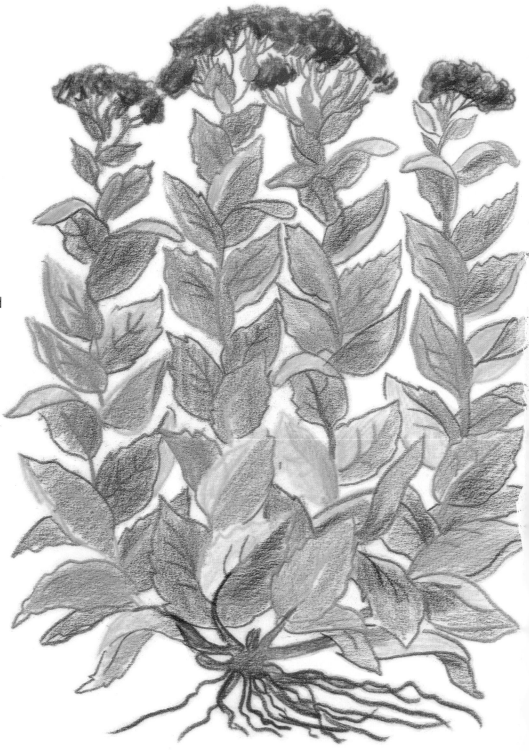

**Lawsonia (henna) plant**

## The Advantages of Using 100 Percent Natural Henna

Henna is, in many ways, the ideal colorant. Chemically based dyes often cause split ends and lifeless hair; henna conditions. Rather than permeating the hair, henna coats the hair shaft, preventing brittleness and breakage. And because it coats, it wears off gradually over a period of twelve weeks, eliminating the dark-root problem you must contend with when using chemical tints.

Henna highlights and brightens; it gives hair body, texture, and bounce; it helps make hair more manageable; it neutralizes excessive oiliness; and it can be used to beautify *any* type of hair—virgin, tinted, bleached, or streaked. (It actually helps counteract the damaging effects of chemicals on your hair.) Plus, it can be used over and over; each time you rehenna you will be rewarded with deeper color, more body, more sheen.

In fact, just about the only thing henna can't do is transform a brunette into a blonde—henna brightens, but it doesn't lighten. But when henna makes you fall in love with your hair color again, a dramatic two-process change may be the furthest thing from your mind.

## Henna Is More Than Just Red

A popular misconception is that henna means bright red. Actually, today's 100 percent natural henna consists of three basic shades: red, black, and colorless (or natural). It is the combination of these three shades that creates the dazzling array of henna color-enhancers now available:

**Natural** is neutral; it adds shine and highlights to any hair color, including gray.

**Hazel** is perfect for filling in gray or salt-and-pepper hair with dusty-blonde highlights.

**Champagne** is a delicate blonde shade; use it to add a pale blonde glow to blonde, dirty blonde, or light brown hair.

**Cognac** adds beautiful warm honey-red tones to medium brown hair.

**Strawberry blonde** is a golden-red dazzler; it's used as a filler for gray hair and adds reddish-gold highlights to blonde, light brown, and medium brown hair.

**Mahogany** adds warm golden-brown highlights with a hint of red to medium brown hair.

**Brown** is a true chestnut shade, without a trace of red; it brings rich, brown highlights to brown and black hair.

**Red** is a deep-red enhancer for brown and black hair; it's definitely not the flaming-red henna of old.

**Copper** is a rich red-gold highlighter for brown, black, and red hair.

**Auburn** is a red-brown shade that warms up brown, black, and red hair.

**Burgundy** is red-black; it brings out deep-wine highlights in brown or black hair.

**Black** is a deep ebony, adding jet highlights and lots of shine to black hair.

Each of these shades will look slightly different on you than on anyone else; henna works subtly, bringing out the best in your natural hair color. Of course, if you're adventurous, each of these colors can be mixed with others to create new shades: a blend of two parts red and one part burgundy, for example, will result in a plum shade. But for the majority of women (particularly those not experienced in applying henna), one of the twelve shades described above will do just fine.

# When Applying Henna

- **You may need preconditioning.** If your hair is bleached or unusually dry, using a henna conditioner before you add color will enable your hair to get the maximum benefit—maximum sheen and maximum body—from henna. And because henna coats the hair, it will lock in the moisture of your conditioner.

- **Make sure hair is dry.** Henna is most effectively applied to dry hair. If hair needs washing, shampoo and *dry* before applying henna.

- **Brush hair briskly** to get dust and leftover hair spray out of the hair. Otherwise, color won't "take" properly.

- **It may be easier to work with a partner** at least the first time around. Although henna application is really not that complicated, your reach may exceed your grasp; application could be uneven.

- **Timing is a key.** The longer you leave henna on your hair, the more intense and dramatic the final shade will be. The shorter the application, the more your natural hair color will shine through.

    The following color chart offers suggestions for the best results.

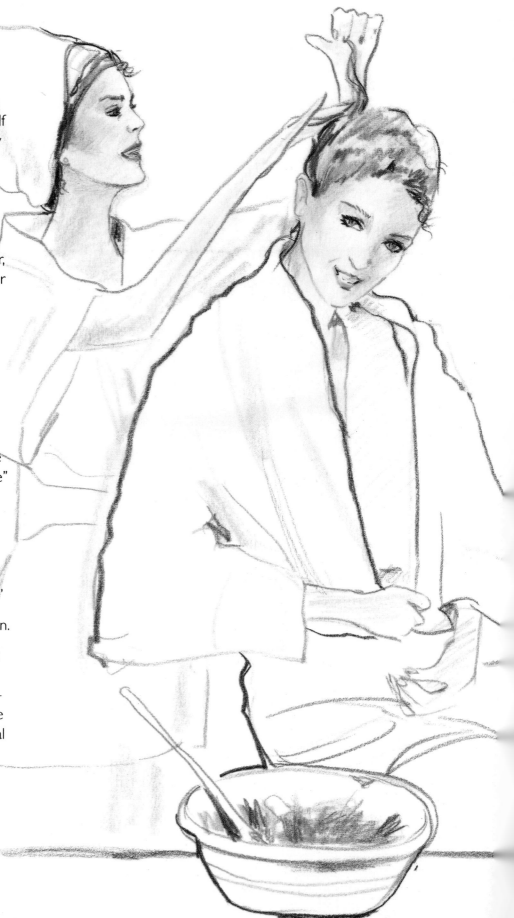

# Henna Color Chart

| If Your Hair Color Is: | Natural | Hazel | Champagne | Strawberry Blonde | Cognac | Mahogany | Brown | Red | Copper | Auburn | Burgundy | Black |
|---|---|---|---|---|---|---|---|---|---|---|---|---|
| **Blonde** | 45 MIN. | 45 MIN. | 35 MIN. | 25 MIN. | | 45 MIN.* | | 30 MIN. | 1 HOUR* | 45 MIN.* | | |
| **Strawberry Blonde** | 45 MIN. | 1 HOUR | 25 MIN. | 1 HOUR | 45 MIN. | 45 MIN.* | | 45 MIN. | 1 HOUR | 45 MIN. | | |
| **Light Brown** | 45 MIN. | 1 HOUR | 45 MIN. | 25 MIN. | 45 MIN. | 1 HOUR | 1 HOUR* | ½ HOUR | 1 HOUR* | 1 HOUR* | | |
| **Dark Brown** | 45 MIN. | 1 HOUR | | | 1 HOUR | 1 HOUR | 1 HOUR | 45 MIN. | 1 HOUR | 1 HOUR | 2 HOURS | 2 HOURS |
| **Red** | 45 MIN. | 1 HOUR | | | 1 HOUR | | 45 MIN. | 1 HOUR | 1 HOUR | 1 HOUR | 1½ HOURS | 1½ HOURS |
| **Black** | 45 MIN. | | | | 1 HOUR | 1 HOUR | 1 HOUR | 2 HOURS | | 2 HOURS | 1½ HOURS | 1 HOUR |
| **50% Gray** | 45 MIN. | 45 MIN. | 30 MIN. | 30 MIN. | 1 HOUR* | 1 HOUR* | 1 HOUR* | 1 HOUR | 1 HOUR* | 1 HOUR* | 1 HOUR* | 1 HOUR* |
| **100% Gray** | 45 MIN. | 30 MIN. | 35 MIN. | 20 MIN. | | | | | | | | |

**The Basic Henna Shades**

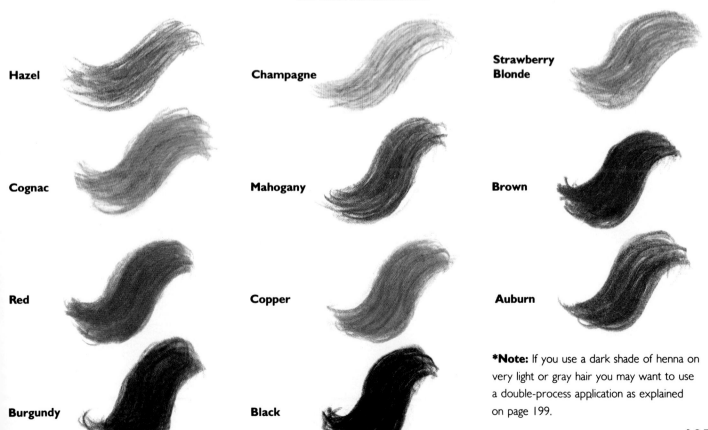

Hazel

Champagne

Strawberry Blonde

Cognac

Mahogany

Brown

Red

Copper

Auburn

Burgundy

Black

**\*Note:** If you use a dark shade of henna on very light or gray hair you may want to use a double-process application as explained on page 199.

195

## Applying Henna
## Step-By-Step

**1.** Your materials—henna, a non-metallic mixing bowl, a wooden or plastic spoon, rubber gloves, aluminum foil, boiling water, and shampoo. (Also, keep a clock or watch handy.)

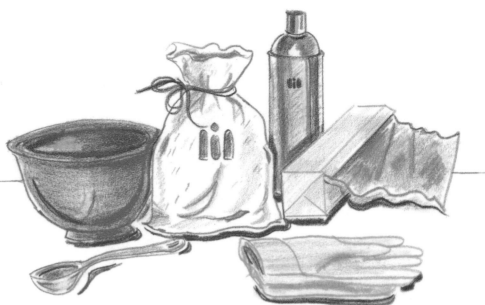

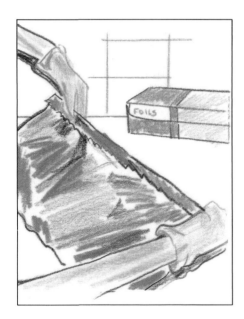

**2.** Cut off a piece of foil the length of your arm, fold edge over so it won't scratch your neck, and put aside until after application.

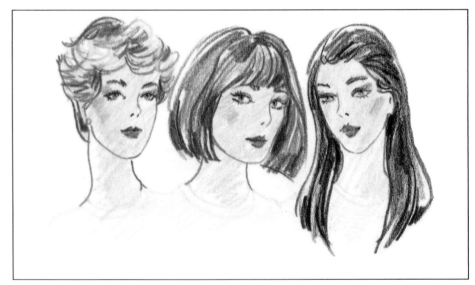

**3.** For fine, short hair, use 2½ ounces or 5 heaping tablespoons of henna; for fine, shoulder-length hair, use 4 ounces or 8 heaping tablespoons; for thick, shoulder-length hair, use 8 ounces or 16 heaping tablespoons; for very long or very thick hair, more henna may be necessary.

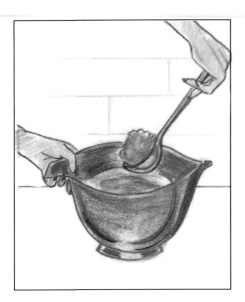

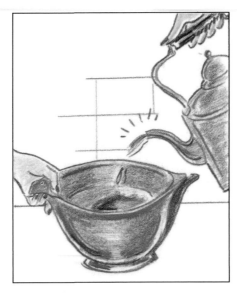

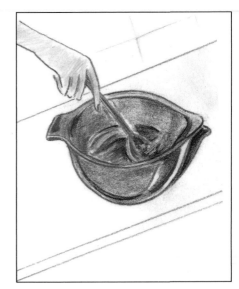

**4.** Put henna in a bowl. Add boiling water gradually, stirring (as though mixing dough) until the

mixture reaches the consistency of sour cream. Proper mixing is very important—

mix thoroughly for at least five to seven minutes.

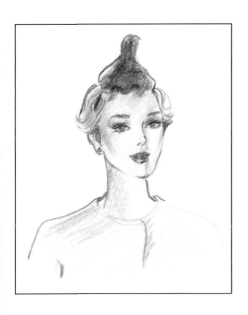

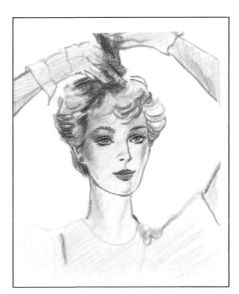

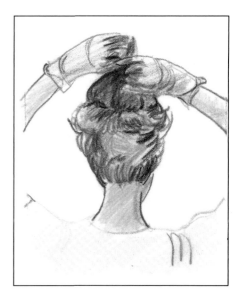

**5.** After putting on gloves (you'll need them to prevent staining unless you're using natural, colorless henna), apply mixture to dry, unwashed hair. Always work over a sink. Start application at the crown of the head.

**6.** Work in an ever-widening circular direction.

**7.** After henna has been applied to each section, place hair close to crown.

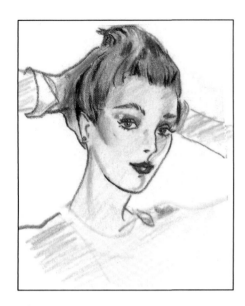

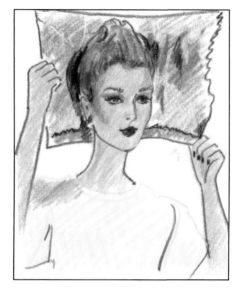

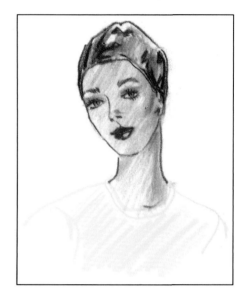

**8.** Keep hair close to the head after applying henna to avoid any mess. Then massage henna into the hair, working from the nape of the neck to the crown, until hair is evenly covered.

**9.** Wrap head with aluminum foil to seal in natural body heat. For best results, henna should remain on the hair for time recommended in the color chart.

**10.** External heat from a heat lamp, hot dryer, or cap, cuts by half the time of application; use a plastic cap, *not* aluminum foil, with external heat.

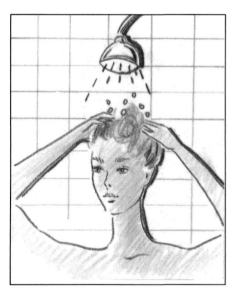

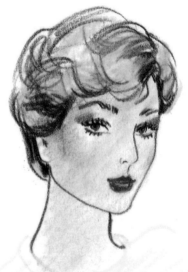

**11.** Unwrap head; rinse thoroughly with warm water to remove henna from hair, then shampoo. After your hair is dry, you will begin to see the difference; your hair will be brighter, shinier, more beautiful. For maximum color and sheen, don't shampoo again for at least twenty-four hours (the henna will continue coating the shaft until then). Color will begin to fade in six weeks; to encourage henna buildup, reapply within four to six weeks even if the color still looks fresh and bright. More henna will only make your hair stronger and more vibrant.

## Single-Process Color for Gray, Bleached, or Naturally Blonde Hair

When going darker, light or gray hair usually requires a double-process, but there are times when blondes and women who are slightly or entirely gray can use a single henna application to boost color and shine.

If you have *less than 10 percent gray hair*, the two henna shades that will work best in a single application are strawberry blonde and mahogany, mixed half and half. After forty-five minutes, hair will be a glowing medium brown touched with rich, red highlights.

To bring out silver highlights in *100 percent gray hair*, use a single-process application of natural henna. Hair will glisten! Or try these other one-step alternatives: hazel, to add glowing, ash-blond highlights, or champagne, which brings a golden-blond gleam to gray hair.

Use single-process hazel or champagne henna to highlight *bleached or naturally blonde* hair, as well.

---

### For Instant Highlights

You can change your hair color as easily as you change your makeup and your mood if you keep henna styling gels on hand. Just sweep on and comb through for rich color that highlights your face, strengthens your hair—then washes out completely with your next shampoo.

---

## Important— If You Use a Temporary Rinse

Temporary rinses do not allow henna to coat hair; instead, they both block the henna and mix with it during shampooing, causing streaking and uneven color. To ensure good results, be sure to wash a temporary rinse out completely before applying henna to hair.

## Double-Process Color for Gray or Light Hair

If you have light hair and want to make it darker, or if your hair is heavily pepper-and-salt, you must use a double-process henna application. Dark shades do not color light hair evenly unless the hair has been prepared first with a red-tinted henna filler shade.

### First Process

If your hair is gray with a light color base, or if you want your light hair to remain light, use strawberry blonde henna, leaving it on your hair for twenty-five minutes. If your hair is gray with a dark color base, or if you are preparing your hair to go darker, use red henna, leaving it on for forty-five minutes.

After the first process, rinse your hair thoroughly (but don't shampoo), and blow it dry.

### Second Process

Apply the henna shade you desire and leave it on *twice as long* as the first application. The extra time allows your final shade to cover the filler tint completely. Rinse thoroughly, shampoo—and look fabulous!

# Putting It All Together in a Day of Beauty

If you have adopted my program for super skin as the basis of your daily complexion ritual, if you have begun to experiment with the exciting, dramatic makeups that can fill your life with color, you are looking and feeling more beautiful already. But even if you have yet to open the door to your beauty potential, waiting to pick up a fluff brush until after you've put down this book, as long as you have begun to think about yourself in a fresh, new way you have reason to *celebrate*. The many looks of you—and the techniques that can unlock your unique beauty—are within your reach. Why not really *revel* in what makes you so special by treating yourself to a salon-quality day of beauty? Invest just one pampering,

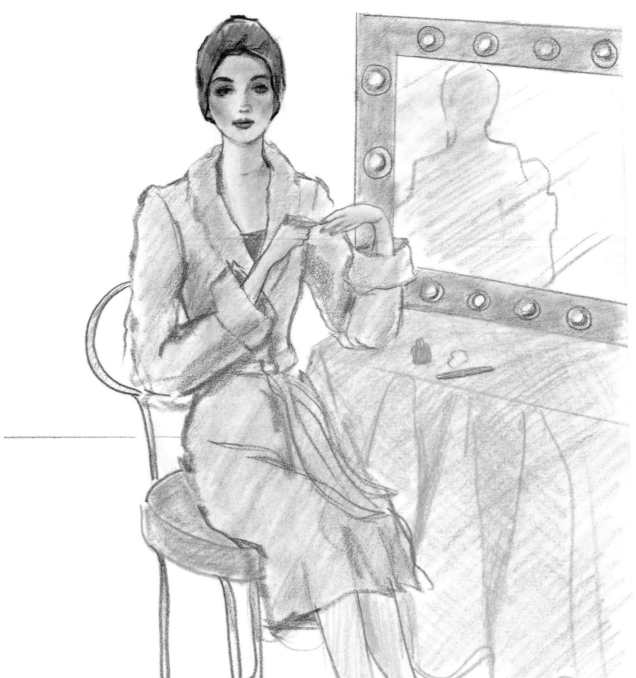

revitalizing afternoon in your most important asset
—yourself—and the beauty dividends you will reap will
go more than skin-deep. So splurge—turn your home
into a luxurious spa and polish your look to a healthy
glow. You're worth it!

# **T**IME OUT

This is *your* time to luxuriate in solitude—and give yourself a big beauty boost by starting off with a deep henna-conditioning treatment to make hair shine. Slather it on—then, while the conditioner penetrates, treat yourself to a twenty-minute minifacial to get your skin glowing. Start with a deep-cleaning scrub, then apply your favorite mask. By the time the mask has loosened surface debris and dead cells, you'll be ready to rinse away the mask and the henna in an invigorating shower. You'll emerge revitalized. And because your shower has gently steamed your pores, your skin will be primed to accept the moisturizing benefits of an allover skin treat—the five-minute moisturizer massage. Finish with a manicure and pedicure, and you're relaxed, pampered, and polished, ready to admire the effects of your head-to-toe spa treatments. Just don't be surprised when others admire them, too!

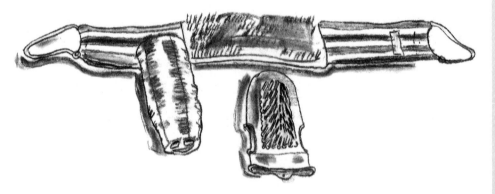

**Massage your body with a natural loofah to bring out your skin's natural glow.**

# **T**HE FRENCH MANICURE

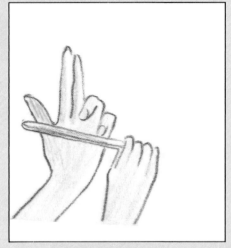

**1.** File nails in one direction only to make sure the tips are smooth.

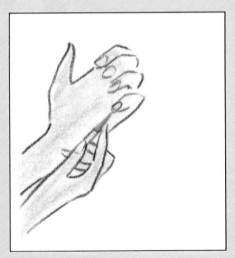

**2.** Use a white pencil under the nail tips to give them a clean, shining look.

# **T**HE PEDICURE

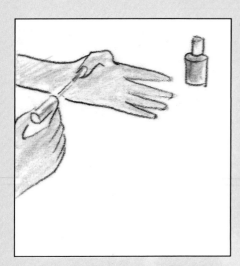

**3.** Carefully apply white opaque enamel to the tips and let it dry. Then cover the entire nail with a coat of sheer pink polish. After it dries, finish with a clear top coat.

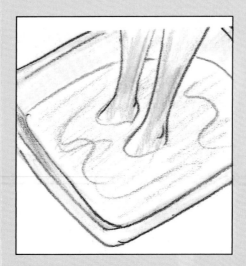

**1.** When it comes to beautifying and pampering your feet, nothing beats a pedicure.

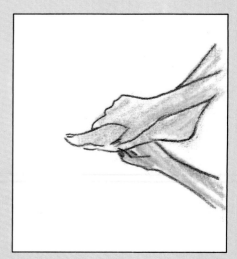

**2.** Massage your feet to relax and revitalize them. Apply pressure all over the bottoms of your feet with your thumb.

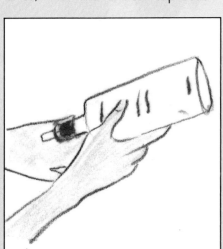

**4.** Treat yourself to a two-minute miosturizing hand massage.

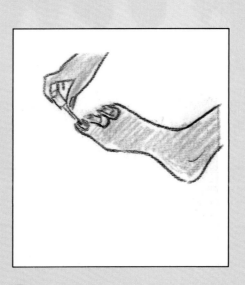

**3.** Twist a tissue and wrap it between your toes to separate them. Apply a clear base coat and let it dry. Finish with one or two coats of color polish, brushing from base of nail to tip.

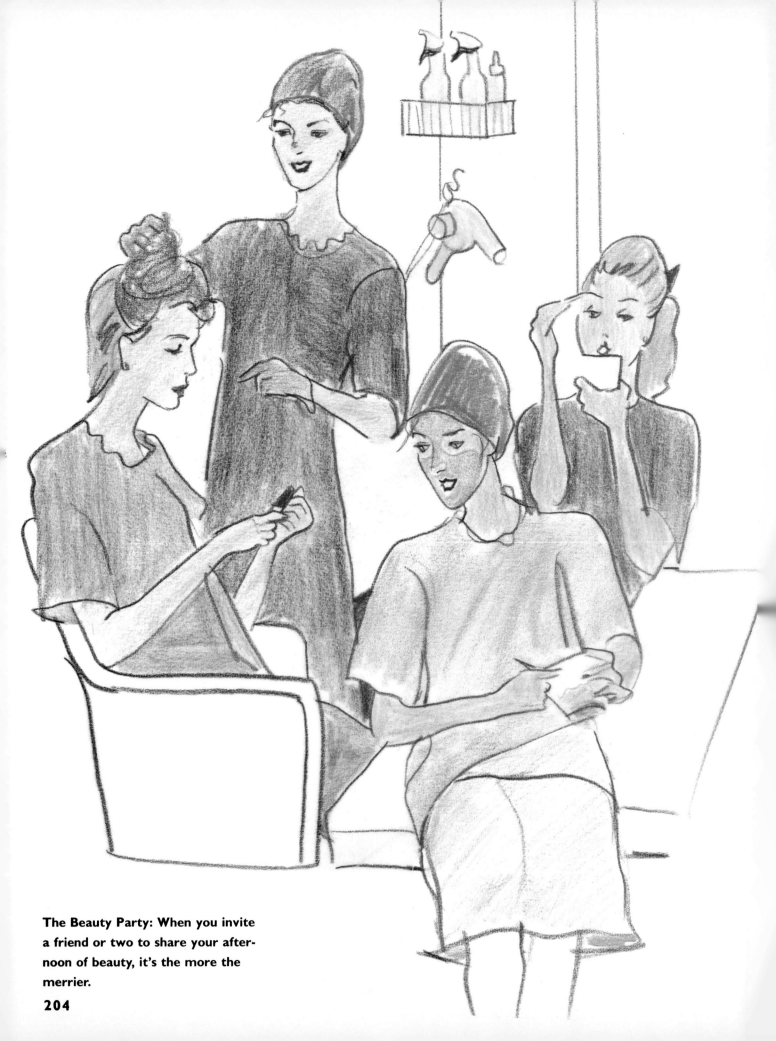

**The Beauty Party:** When you invite a friend or two to share your afternoon of beauty, it's the more the merrier.

204

# IF I'VE MADE YOU FEEL BEAUTIFUL…

I hope you'll let me know. Helping women to put their best faces forward is more than my career—it is my continued ambition. When do *I* feel beautiful? When a woman looks in the mirror and recognizes her uniqueness through my handiwork.

Put my skin-saving strategies to work for you. Experiment with color to bring out your special characteristics. You'll feel confident, energized—*beautiful*. But that was my promise to you, wasn't it?

# Credits, The Many Looks of You

Model: Caroline Reid
Agency: Legends, NYC
Evening (car): Snakeskin jacket from New York Fashion Club, NYC; Jewelry from Y'lang-Y'lang, NYC
Nightplay: Taken at Pronto Ristorante, NYC; Dress from New York Fashion Club, NYC
Hairstylist: Cohl, NYC


Model: Lisa Berkley
Agency: Elite Models, NYC
Evening: White suit from Giorgio Armani; Jewelry from Y'lang-Y'lang, NYC
Nightplay (in limousine): Jewelry from Y'lang-Y'lang, NYC; Fox fur coat from Ritz Thrift Shop, NYC
Hairstylist: Gili Gamliel/il-Makiage, NYC


Model: Jade
Agency: Wilhemina, NYC
Morning (store): Shot on location at Parachute, Los Angeles; Pink suit and hat by Harry Parnass and Nicola Pelly for Parachute, Los Angeles; Jewelry from Connie Parente, Los Angeles
Afternoon: Earrings from Connie Parente, Los Angeles; Shirt from Jones, Beverly Hills/London
Nightplay: Tuxedo jacket by Harry Parnass and Nicola Pelly for Parachute, Los Angeles; White tuxedo shirt from The Big Bang, Los Angeles
Hairstylist: Edward Sanchez of Doyle Wilson Salon, Los Angeles

Model: Debbie Dickinson
Agency: Elite Models, NYC
Morning (in salon): Jewelry from Y'lang-Y'lang, NYC
Evening (bride): Wedding gown from Kleinfeld's, Brooklyn, NY; Jewelry from Y'lang-Y'lang, NYC
Nightplay (gold): Jewelry from Y'lang-Y'lang, NYC
Hairstylist (Morning and Evening): Gili Gamliel/il-Makiage, NYC
Hairstylist (Nightplay): Yamasa of Suga Salon, NYC


Model: Jennifer Gatti
Agency: Elite Models, NYC
Nightplay: Silver Cocoon by Larry Le Gaspi; Earrings by Kenneth J. Lane; Stylist: Pat Kurs, NYC
Hairstylist: Gili Gamliel/il-Makiage, NYC


Model: Zacki Murphy
Agency: Ford Models, NYC
Morning (office): Jewelry from Jaded, NYC
Evening: Floral shirt from Jones, Beverly Hills/London; Necklace from Connie Parente, Los Angeles
Nightplay: Black sequin gown from The Big Bang, Los Angeles; Jewelry from Connie Parente, Los Angeles
Hairstylist (Morning): Ron Lewis of Bruno La Salon, NYC
Hairstylist (Evening and Nightplay): GI Joe of Giuseppe Franco Salon, Beverly Hills

Model: Lisa Hewitt
Agency: Nina Blanchard, CA
Before: Kimono robe, The Big Bang, Los Angeles
Morning (lab): Earrings, Connie Parente, Los Angeles
Evening (safari): Jacket, The Big Bang, Los Angeles
Nightplay: Suit, Jones, Beverly Hills/London; Jewelry, Connie Parente, Los Angeles
Hairstylist: Taylor of Allen Edwards Salon, Beverly Hills


Model: Kersti Bowser
Agency: Elite Models, NYC
Morning (with violin): Violin from "We Buy Guitars Inc.," NYC
Nightplay: Jewelry from Wendy Gell, NYC
Hairstylist: Gili Gamliel/il-Makiage, NYC


Model: Tina Littlewood
Agency: Mary Webb Davis, Los Angeles
Morning (typewriter): Shirt from Emilio Che at Moshi-Moshi, Los Angeles
Nightplay: Red silk jumpsuit by Kathreen Hamnet at Jones, Beverly Hills/London

**Makeup for all nine models by Ilana Harkavi/il-Makiage, NYC**

**Stylist: Miss Lola Ehrhart, Los Angeles/NYC (for all shots except Nightplay, Jennifer Gatti)**

**Stylist for Powder Room photo taken at the Paladium, NYC (p. 78–79): Pat Kurs**